WHEN THE DOCTOR SAYS IT'S INFERTILITY, THIS POSITIVE
APPROACH EMPOWERS YOU TO FIND ANSWERS AND TAKE ACTION

A diagnosis of infertility may leave you feeling heartbroken,
angry, or helpless. More than just a medical condition, being
infertile touches deep emotional chords within both men and
women, having an impact on self-esteem, sexuality, and family relationships. But as this upbeat, positive guide stresses,
infertile means "pre-pregnant." Medical technology, genetic
testing, and strides in understanding the role of stress in preventing conception have created an array of new treatment
options that can result in the pregnancy you desire. Whether
it's the facts about which women benefit from vitamin B-6
supplementation, suggested exercises for those feeling pressured by sex-on-demand, or the cost of the latest hi-tech procedures, this must-have book brings real help to infertile
couples.

50 ESSENTIAL THINGS TO DO
WHEN THE DOCTOR SAYS
IT'S INFERTILITY

B. BLAKE LEVITT is an award-winning medical and science
writer. A member of the American Medical Writers Associa-
tion, the National Association of Science Writers, the Author's
Guild and the Author's League, she is the co-author of *Before
You Conceive, The Complete Prepregnancy Guide*, written with
John R. Sussman, M.D., for which she won the Will Solimene
Book Award for Excellence in Medical Communication. She
lives in Warren, Connecticut.

50

ESSENTIAL THINGS TO DO WHEN THE DOCTOR SAYS IT'S INFERTILITY

B. BLAKE LEVITT

AN AUTHORS GUILD BACKINPRINT.COM EDITION

50 Essential Things To Do
When The Doctor Says It's Infertility
All Rights Reserved © 1995, 2000 by B. Blake Levitt

AN AUTHORS GUILD BACKINPRINT.COM EDITION

Published by iUniverse.com, Inc.

For information address:
iUniverse.com, Inc.
620 North 48th Street, Suite 201
Lincoln, NE 68504-3467
www.iuniverse.com

Originally published by Plume/Penguin

ISBN: 0-595-09235-7

Printed in the United States of America

To My Mom,
Who gave me the greatest gift she could . . .
Life.

CONTENTS

PART ONE

WHAT INFERTILITY IS

INTRODUCTION:
UNDERSTANDING INFERTILITY

Up until the time you decide to have a baby, most of your energy concerning the subject of fertility has probably gone into preventing conception. People simply assume their contraception methods are working when, in fact, they may be experiencing impaired fertility. Infertility has risen sharply in the last ten years, and everyone seems to know someone who is having difficulty conceiving. It is estimated that between 10 and 18 percent of the reproductive population in the United States is infertile at any given time. There are several explanations for the problem, including women delaying pregnancy until after age twenty-five, when their less fertile years begin; an increase in sexual activity in general along with the advent of the Pill for women and the accompanying disuse of condoms in men—all of which lead to the spread of venereal infections; and the widespread exposure to a variety of environmental toxins.

Popularly defined as the inability to become pregnant after one year or more of regular sexual activity without contraception, or as the inability to carry a pregnancy through to the live birth of a baby, infertility is considered common today. Approximately half of the couples trying to conceive will do so within three to five months, depending on whether they already have children, another 25 percent within six months, and an additional 5 to 10 percent within a year. But one out of every six couples is infertile at any given time.

Infertility is described as *primary* when pregnancy has never occurred, and *secondary* when a couple has had at least one child but cannot seem to conceive again. *Sterility* is the absolute inability to conceive. When the fertility of one or both spouses is reduced, the couple is *subfertile.* Subfertile individuals may be capable of conceiving easily with partners whose fertility is enhanced. For example, a man with a low sperm count may be able to father a child more easily with a woman who ovulates more than once within a menstrual cycle. And a woman with irregular ovulation may be able to conceive more easily (when she does ovulate) with a man with a very high sperm count.

There are many frustrating gray areas regarding infertility. Things are often not as black and white as we would like, and therefore aren't easily solvable. It is not unusual for a doctor to treat both partners in cases of subfertility—such as prescribing fertility medication for the spouse of a man with a low sperm count—in an effort to increase pregnancy possibilities for the couple.

Peak fertility for women occurs in their mid-twenties. Fertility declines gradually until age thirty, and then begins to drop more rapidly. Women in their thirties who are having difficulty conceiving should seek help quickly. Fertility for men decreases gradually from the teenage years onward. Rates of conception for men age forty are about one-third those of men under age twenty-five.

Aspects of your general and reproductive health history have a significant bearing on your ability to become pregnant. The birth control methods you use, sexually transmitted diseases, undiagnosed urinary tract infections, hormonal imbalances, abortions done under unsterile conditions, miscarriages, uterine abnormalities, previous adverse obstetrical experiences, and genetically transmitted disorders can affect the pregnancy process, including your ability to become pregnant in the first place. Women with irregular menstrual cycles may not be ovulating regularly and may need treatment in order to conceive. Men who contracted mumps during their adult years, or women with a history of pelvic inflammatory disease, may want to forgo delays in starting or adding to their families since these conditions may impair fertility.

Many infertile couples conceive. Many do not. A number of things can have a positive influence on your experience, especially attitude. Infertility by definition is *pre*pregnant. Thinking of yourself as *infertile* sometimes lays a shroud of defectiveness over you and your mate. Try thinking of yourself as prepregnant instead.

Disappointment, frustration, and negativity are common feelings for an infertile couple. The purpose of this book is to focus on the positive, however, and to help you take a proactive role in understanding and dealing with infertility.

1

FIND AN INFERTILITY SPECIALIST

The first and most important thing for you to do is to find a good specialist. You must be under the care of a trained infertility specialist who understands the often subtle complexities that affect fertility. Sometimes the causes are obvious. Other times their discovery calls for a medical mystery hunt.

Not all OB-GYNs specialize in infertility. If infertility assessment and treatment are mere additions to a long list of OB-GYN services on a particular doctor's roster, keep looking until you find someone with a genuine concentration in the subject. Most OB-GYNs today have access to sperm banks and can do in vitro fertilization in their offices, but this does *not* make these practitioners infertility specialists.

There are specific qualifications for a subspecialty in infertility, including a two-year fellowship in reproductive endocrinology. Infertility can be extremely complex, and so it is important for you to find someone who really knows his or her way around it. Look for a board-certified infertility specialist or reproductive endocrinologist.

Start your search with personal referrals. Do you know anyone who has had impaired fertility? Find out what they did, who they consulted, and what the results were both medically and emotionally. Nurses at your local hospital are also good sources of information, and many major teaching hospitals have infertility clinics. Your county or state medical society may also be able to provide information on doctors with infertility subspecialties. Ask for referrals in your area.

The Yellow Pages are another resource. Doctors usually list their areas of expertise in the "Physicians" section. Group practices with several physicians under one roof may have one or two doctors who specialize in infertility. Be sure to check any name you get through the phone book with a national organization such as Resolve, Inc., or the American Fertility Society.

Be wary of solo practitioners who list every OB-GYN service under the sun. It is unlikely that any doctor in a solo practice has the time to fully concentrate on obstetrics and infertility at the same time, despite what he or she advertises.

You may already have a gynecologist that you like a great deal and want to keep. Depending on how old you are and how long you've been trying to conceive, this attitude may be more sentimental than wise. Try to set a deadline in your mind beyond which you will seek other help if pregnancy hasn't occurred. There is nothing wrong with shopping around. You're hiring the doctor, not vice versa. And it is generally recommended that you get a second opinion, even if you stay with your regular OB-GYN.

Here are the addresses and phone numbers of three national organizations that can provide information on infertility specialists in your area. Include a self-addressed, stamped envelope when you write.

The American Society for Reproductive Medicine
1209 Montgomery Highway
Birmingham, AL 35216
(205) 978-5000

The American College of Obstetricians and Gynecologists
600 Maryland Avenue, SW
Suite 300 East
Washington, DC 20024
(202) 638-5577

Resolve, Inc.
1310 Broadway
Somerville, MA 02144
(617) 623-0744

Look for a doctor whose practice is made up of at least 50 percent infertility work. When you make your inquiry phone calls, ask the receptionist about how much of the doctor's patient roster is devoted to infertility cases. Have patients given their permission to be contacted by prospective clients? For balance, you also should ask for the names of people who haven't conceived successfully.

Try to set up preliminary interviews with several doctors. If possible, both partners should attend these meetings since you may be working with this person for a long time. It's important that all of you feel equally comfortable. Have a list of questions ready. Here are some things to find out:

- Is the doctor board certified in reproductive endocrinology? (To receive board certification, the doctor must have completed his or her fellowship and passed both the written and oral exams for reproductive endocrinology.)
- How long has the doctor specialized in infertility? How many patients does the doctor currently treat? What are the success rates? Does the doctor have any special training in the field? (Special training can sometimes offset a shorter time in private practice.)
- Does the doctor do surgical procedures? What special training has he or she had? Does that person have a particular approach to infertility? Why? What are the success rates?

(For example, success rates for microsurgery procedures should be 60 percent or better.)

- What are the doctor's own resources? Does he or she use one main laboratory that specializes in fertility work? (Dividing up the many samples necessary and sending them to various labs takes more time and costs a lot more.) Does the doctor use one main hospital for infertility cases? (Using only one hospital is better because it's more likely you'll get specialized treatment.)

- Does the doctor use drug therapy to induce ovulation? If so, what is it and how is follow-up done? What are the risks? What are the pregnancy rates? (Pregnancy rates can range between 2 and 70 percent, depending on which fertility drugs are used and why they are prescribed. Ask what is "normal" to expect.)

- What happens if pregnancy doesn't occur? Can the doctor refer you to adoption agencies? genetics counselors? support groups?

- How did you and your mate react emotionally to the doctor? Did you feel rushed? Spoken down to? Was the doctor truly forthcoming and willing to give you information, or did he or she hold all the cards close to the chest, expecting you to automatically trust their authority?

AN IMPORTANT THING YOU CAN DO

Contact the infertility groups mentioned in this chapter and get the names of specialists in your area.

#2

Know What to Expect from an Infertility Workup

Couples who have had intercourse without contraceptives twice a week for a year without becoming pregnant will undoubtedly be referred for infertility counseling. This kind of counseling is time-consuming, energy-draining, and expensive, and it will delve into the most personal aspects of your lives. It is best not to begin this process unless you are committed to following it through to a definite answer as to why you are unable to become pregnant. If you don't pursue this course to the end, you will still be wondering years down the road.

Both partners need to participate. Many of the questions will be extremely personal and may embarrass some people. But keep in mind that counselors ask these questions to help you overcome infertility.

Couples should expect to answer questions about the following:

- Each partner's family history, to detect any genetic disorders

- Each partner's health history, with special attention given to diseases that have an impact on fertility, such as diabetes, mumps, rubella, thyroid and glandular disorders, and tuberculosis, as well as some other infections
- Medications, both over-the-counter and prescription
- The couple's lifestyle, including intake of alcohol, drugs, coffee, and tea; cigarette smoking; and recreational activities (for example, participation in sports that require men to wear athletic supports, or using hot tubs or saunas)
- The female partner's sexual history: when menstruation began, what menstrual periods are like, pain experienced between periods, previous pregnancies, miscarriages, past surgery, abortions, pain during intercourse, venereal or pelvic infections, use of lubricants such as Vaseline, use of contraceptives and spermicides, and number of sex partners
- The male partner's sexual history: normal descent of the testicles, past surgery, circumcision (and at what age), injuries to the testicles, venereal infections, contraceptive methods, and number of sex partners
- The couple's sexual behavior: frequency of intercourse, orgasmic patterns, preferred positions, masturbation, and any other sexual techniques

In addition to answering the above questions, the female partner will be taught to take and record her basal body temperature each morning when she wakes to help determine if and when she is ovulating, and both partners will undergo extensive physical examinations, including blood and other laboratory tests. Couples will also follow three essential phases in an infertility workup, all of which can be completed within two months.

PHASE 1: Specialists look for the most readily available answers to infertility at this stage. The main evaluation is done now, as are blood work and the basic physical. Also included in Phase 1 is a postcoital test, usually done two to four hours after intercourse, which samples cervical mucus in a routine pelvic examination. This answers such important questions as: Is there enough estrogen? Are the sperm motile? What is the pH and consistency of the cervical mucus?

Blood tests are done to determine if either partner has a hormonal imbalance. A basal body temperature chart (see #33) will come in handy to indicate the woman's ovulatory patterns. Sperm analysis will also be done to determine size, shape, motility, and number of sperm, as well as the amount of seminal fluid. Any persistent abnormalities indicate the need for further evaluation of the male partner by a urologist.

By the end of Phase 1, the problem may be traced to ovulation, sperm characteristics, cervical mucus disorders, or hormonal imbalances.

PHASE 2: If Phase 1 provides no answers to the cause of infertility, it will be recommended that the anatomical structure of the woman's fallopian tubes and endometrium be examined for causes. In Phase 2 doctors recommend a hysterosalpingogram (HSG), also called a tubogram or uterogram. During this test, which is an outpatient procedure, an iodine dye is inserted through the cervix into the uterus and fallopian tubes. The dye is then traced with X ray to determine any blockages or irregularities in the uterus or tubes. To evaluate the uterine lining, the endometrium is biopsied to find out if it is responding properly to hormonal stimulation. If antisperm antibodies are suspected, tests are done for confirmation. Keeping your basal body temperature chart will continue to be recommended.

Another diagnostic tool that may be recommended during Phase 2 is called a hysteroscope, a fiberoptic tube inserted through the cervix into the uterus, which allows the doctor to see the uterus and fallopian tube connections directly. This test can be done in a hospital or under local anesthesia in a doctor's office. It is useful for detecting uterine scar tissue and uterine irregularities, such as polyps, fibroids, and membrane walls (septa), which can cause infertility.

If the male partner's sperm was found to be abnormal in the Phase 1 evaluation, Phase 2 might include a testicular biopsy, which can be done at an outpatient surgi-center or in a hospital.

By the end of Phase 2, the existence of physical blockages to the uterus and fallopian tubes, as well as testicular disorders, will either be confirmed or eliminated as causes of infertility.

PHASE 3: If no satisfactory answers are yet forthcoming, Phase 3 requires a direct surgical look into the woman's abdominal cavity at the ovaries, fallopian tubes, and uterus, and for abnormal endometrial tissue growth (endometriosis). A laparoscopy, done in the hospital under anesthesia, involves the doctor inserting a small lighted tube through the abdominal area to view the reproductive organs. A hysteroscopy, utilizing a similar lighted fiberoptic tube inserted through the cervix directly into the uterus, may also be recommended. Basal body temperature continues to be important to record.

Men who have varicoceles (varicose veins in the penis), which cause poor sperm production, or any blockages to the epididymis, vas deferens, urethra, or ejaculatory ducts (all parts of the male reproductive system) will already have been recommended for corrective surgery by Phase 3.

By the end of Phase 3, all aspects of each partner's reproductive system should have been comprehensively evaluated and treatment recommended. In some cases, however, the causes of infertility remain unknown. It doesn't mean that the causes are unknowable, but that at the present state of infertility technology no diagnosis can be made.

AN IMPORTANT THING YOU CAN DO

Have all of your medical records and histories available for both partners. Try to think of any genetic disorders that might run in your families.

PART TWO

UNDERSTAND THE PHYSIOLOGY OF FEMALE INFERTILITY

#3

KNOW WHAT CAUSES INFERTILITY IN WOMEN

Infertility in women is far better studied than it is in men. Here are nine things that can impair a woman's ability to conceive:

1. Menstrual cycle irregularities and hormonal imbalances
2. Ovarian disorders
3. Corpus luteum disorders
4. Fallopian tube disorders
5. Uterine disorders
6. Cervical mucus disorders
7. Habitual miscarriage
8. Exposure to diethylstilbestrol (DES)
9. Sexual dysfunction

AN IMPORTANT THING YOU CAN DO

Find out if your mother took any medication while she was carrying you. DES could have been prescribed if she or her doctor had any reason to suspect that she might miscarry.

#4

GET TO KNOW YOUR
MENSTRUAL CYCLES

A woman's monthly menstrual cycle is an intricate act of hormonal balance based on general good health. Any number of things can disrupt the process, which in turn can adversely affect fertility. Knowing what is "normal" for you will help you to identify any subtle changes that may have an impact on fertility.

THE "AVERAGE" MENSTRUAL CYCLE

On average, women in the United States have their first period (menarche) at the age of 12.6 years. This age has been decreasing by three to four months per decade over the last century, probably due to better hygiene and nutrition. However, early menstruation is predominantly hereditary.

Most women experience menarche when they are between nine and seventeen years old. Factors that delay the onset of menstruation include poor nutrition; heredity; severe illnesses, such as rheumatic fever and diabetes; mental illness; eating disorders like anorexia nervosa; and severe emotional shock or great stress during puberty. Some lifestyle factors also delay or stop menstruation, including extreme physical exercise, such as training for marathon runners, and living at high altitudes. Light also seems to affect it. Blind females tend to menstruate earlier. Neither race nor climate appears to affect menarche.

A normal cycle ranges between twenty and forty days; the average is twenty-eight days. Normal menstrual flow lasts between one and seven days. Women establish their own life-long individual cycles (usually within the first few years of menstruation) that become "normal" for them. For example, some women have twenty-two-day cycles with a four-day flow and others have thirty-five-day cycles with a six-day flow. The amount of menstrual flow also differs from person to person.

Changes in the length of your cycle of a few days in either direction and different amounts of menstrual flow are common. Small variations do not mean that you have irregular periods.

IRREGULAR MENSTRUAL CYCLES

Irregular periods are common in both young women just beginning to menstruate and women approaching menopause. This is because they may not be ovulating (releasing eggs) regularly but are still producing estrogen. It is the production of estrogen without ovulation that leads to irregular periods since ovulation itself determines the time when the uterus sloughs off its endometrial lining, resulting in menstruation. The endometrial growth in each cycle is stimulated by the production of estrogen within the ovaries.

If your cycle has been regular, and suddenly you experience very painful menstruation (dysmenorrhea), profuse or prolonged bleeding, erratic cycles or failure to menstruate (amenorrhea), this may signal other, more serious, illnesses. You may need a complete physical examination, not just a gynecological checkup.

Irregular periods can be caused by hypo- and hyperthyroidism (under- and overactive thyroid gland, respectively); diabetes; crash dieting and poor nutrition; extreme weight loss or gain; severe emotional stress; tumors of the ovaries, uterus, pituitary gland or hypothalamus; and hormonal imbalances.

From your mid-thirties onward, you may experience slight variations in the degree of menstrual flow and increased symptoms of premenstrual syndrome. And you may not ovulate faithfully within each cycle. Consult your doctor about any drastic changes (the sooner the better) when you are trying to become pregnant, since these changes may indicate problems with your fertility.

AN IMPORTANT THING YOU CAN DO

Keep track of your menstrual cycles on a calendar for several months. Unusual alterations will be apparent within five to six months.

#5

Understand the Rise and Fall of Hormones During Your Menstrual Cycle

Hormones are natural chemicals produced in one part of the body (glands) that flow through the bloodstream and cause changes in other parts of the body. The word *hormone* derives from the Greek *hormōn*, meaning to stir up or set in motion. Products of the endocrine (chemical glandular) system, hormones are responsible for governing the menstrual cycle, the body's metabolism, sexual maturation, the pregnancy process, and many other aspects of our basic physiology.

Understanding your hormonal cycle will help you to identify any changes that might have a negative impact on your fertility. The menstrual cycle is governed by six hormones that work in a tandem chain reaction. These hormones rise and fall during various times of the month along the hormonal axis. (The model that follows is based on a 28-day cycle.)

- *Estrogen* is produced mostly by the ovaries and is primarily responsible for a woman's physiological sexual development. It dominates the first fourteen days of the menstrual cycle and is responsible for stimulating the growth of the endometrium (the lining of the uterus). Estrogen causes an increase in the number of glands and tissue ducts in the breast. In the fallopian tubes, estrogen stimulates the growth of *cilia*, hairlike tissues that push the sperm and egg toward each other and then help transport the fertilized egg toward the uterus. It also stimulates the glands at the base of the cervix to secrete mucus that helps lubricate the vagina, making sperm passage easier, as well as protecting the endometrium from infection. At midcycle, when estrogen levels are highest, the pH of the cervical mucus is alkaline, which is the most hospitable environment for sperm survival.

- *Progesterone* is also produced by the ovaries and dominates the latter half of the menstrual cycle, after ovulation occurs. It thickens the endometrium and promotes cilia growth in the fallopian tubes. (Both estrogen and progesterone stimulate increased mucus production and muscle contractions in the fallopian tubes. The strong stabbing pain some women experience on either side of the abdomen at midcycle may be due to such contractions. This pain is called *mittelschmerz*, which is German for "pain in the middle.") Progesterone also thickens cervical mucus in the latter half of the cycle, chemically changing it to an acidic pH, thereby making the cervix inhospitable to sperm. Furthermore, progesterone slows the growth of the vaginal lining that estrogen stimulated, and is responsible for breast swelling and tenderness.

- *Follicle-stimulating hormone-releasing hormone (FSH-RH)* is produced by the hypothalamus, an area of the lower region of the brain. (The hypothalamus is "central control" for the body's endocrine network, regulating not only the reproductive system but also sexual appetite, hunger, thirst, sleep, and other functions. The hypothalamus reacts sensitively to physical or mental illness. It passes this information on through the hormone system, thereby protecting the menstrual cycle from disorders that have nothing to do with reproductive function.) In the beginning days of the menstrual cycle, estrogen and progesterone are at their lowest levels. The hypothalamus reacts to this by producing FSH-RH, which in turn stimulates the production of FSH in the pituitary gland.

- *Follicle-stimulating hormone (FSH)* is produced in the pituitary gland, which is located below the hypothalamus at the base of the brain. The pituitary gland produces hormones that stimulate many body functions, such as thyroid-stimulating hormone (TSH), which controls basic metabolism; prolactin, which influences milk production; and oxytocin, which induces uterine contractions. FSH stimulates the growth of the ovarian follicles (cell clusters that surround the eggs in the ovary), which in turn produce increasing levels of estrogen and progesterone.
- *Luteinizing hormone-releasing hormone (LH-RH)* is produced in the hypothalamus. At midcycle, when estrogen levels are highest, the hypothalamus responds by producing LH-RH. This triggers the pituitary's production of luteinizing hormone (LH), which then stimulates ovulation.
- *Luteinizing hormone (LH)* is produced by the pituitary in response to LH-RH. It stimulates ovulation. A follicle in the ovary releases an unfertilized egg into the fallopian tube, where it can be fertilized. LH then changes the broken follicle into the *corpus luteum*, which is Latin for "yellow body." After ovulation, the corpus luteum continues to produce high levels of estrogen and progesterone for the next eight to ten days, with progesterone becoming increasingly dominant. The corpus luteum degenerates rapidly toward the end of the cycle, decreasing both estrogen and progesterone levels unless pregnancy has occurred. When the levels fall low enough, the endometrial lining, which has been building up in response to this hormonal interaction, is no longer needed to accommodate a fertilized egg and is sloughed off by the body. Then the cycle begins again.

Hormonal disturbances are responsible for half of all infertility problems in women. Any hitch in this shifting hormonal interaction can interrupt the menstrual cycle and therefore impair fertility. This includes general illness, high fevers, and stress. In fact, a normal, regular menstrual cycle is a sign of general good health, despite how many women have been made to feel about menstruation.

If the hypothalamus fails to respond to low levels of estrogen and does not produce FSH-RH or LH-RH, then the pituitary doesn't get the signal to produce FSH and LH in response, and ovulation doesn't occur—no ovulation, obviously no pregnancy. Common causes are damage to the hypothalamus or pituitary glands, as well as anorexia nervosa and heavy athletic training.

Too much or too little estrogen and progesterone also adversely affect fertility. This can be due to ovarian complications.

Certain medications, especially tranquilizers and mood-altering drugs, can override the hypothalamus and throw off the hormonal cycle enough to disrupt fertility. When the medication is stopped, fertility usually returns.

AN IMPORTANT THING YOU CAN DO

Be aware of your body's normal responses to the ebb and flow of menstrual hormones. When these changes don't occur, be sure to notify your doctor to find out what could be causing the imbalance.

#6

INVESTIGATE FERTILITY DRUGS

Fertility drugs have proved very successful in treating infertility due to hormonal imbalances but have no use in ovulating women suffering infertility from other causes.

There are two basic categories of fertility drugs:

- Clomid and Serophene (clomiphene citrate): Usually, women who are not ovulating lack the midcycle surge of LH produced in the pituitary that triggers ovulation. Generally, these women's bodies produce some estrogen and FSH, but not enough. Clomid, which works directly on the hypothalamus, is an antiestrogen agent and can fool the hypothalamus into thinking that estrogen levels are even lower, thereby causing it to produce more of the FSH-RH that influences the pituitary to produce FSH. FSH then increases the body's estrogen levels. When they reach a certain point, the hypothalamus will produce LH-RH, thereby triggering the pituitary to release LH. Then ovulation can occur. The dose of Clomid may be increased until ovulation occurs.

Taking Clomid will not result in the multiple births reported with the use of other fertility drugs, but there is a 5 to 10 percent increased incidence of having twins if you undergo Clomid therapy.

- Pergonal (HMG) and HCG (gonadotropins): FSH and LH are both *gonadotropins*, a term used to describe reproductive hormones. Sometimes, damage to the hypothalamus or pituitary gland either reduces or eliminates the production of these hormones and causes infertility. It is possible to take these substances directly. Human menopausal gonadotropin (HMG) is a combination of LH and FSH extracted from the urine of menopausal women. (Pergonal is the trade name.) Human chorionic gonadotropin (HCG) is extracted from the urine of pregnant women and is structurally similar to LH. A dose of HCG given at midcycle can stimulate the pituitary's release of LH, thereby producing ovulation.

    Gonadotropin therapy is expensive, needs to be closely monitored with regular estrogen level checks, and is best handled by those with special infertility and endocrinology training. The methods of administering these drugs have greatly improved since their advent. The high incidence of multiple births, while still reported and definitely a risk, has decreased substantially when the therapy is administered by expert hands.

Women seeking solutions for infertility should be very cautious about taking fertility drugs: A handful of recent studies have found a threefold rise in ovarian cancer in women who have taken them. Since only 50 percent of women with ovarian cancer survive five years after being diagnosed, anyone who is at increased risk for the disease—for example, if there is a family history of ovarian cancers—should weigh the risks and benefits *very* carefully before consenting to take these drugs.

Pregnancy itself appears to have a protective effect

against ovarian cancer, so if you become pregnant while taking fertility drugs, any increased risk may be offset by your pregnancy. But research indicates that it isn't a good idea to take fertility drugs indefinitely. And it's possible that doctors will prescribe these drugs less often for the mates of men with low sperm counts.

AN IMPORTANT THING YOU CAN DO

If you are already taking fertility drugs, consider setting a time limit with your doctor.

#7

UNDERSTAND OVARIAN PROBLEMS

There are four basic ovarian abnormalities that can cause infertility in women:

1. Congenital anomalies
2. Benign polycystic ovarian disease, also called Stein-Leventhal syndrome
3. Ovarian tumors
4. Infected ovaries due to pelvic inflammatory disease (PID), gonorrhea, and mumps (See #9, p. 34.)

CONGENITAL ANOMALIES

Sometimes women are born without ovaries or with very small, malformed ones that cannot produce an adequate supply of estrogen or progesterone. Such is the case with Turner's syndrome, a genetically transmitted disorder in which one parent, at the point of conception, does not transfer a necessary X chromosome. Women with Turner's syndrome therefore have only one X chromosome rather than the two X chromosomes needed for normal reproduction.

Turner's syndrome is usually diagnosed in infancy, although sometimes a determination isn't made until puberty, when normal growth and menstruation fail to occur. With estrogen and progesterone therapy, it is possible to promote normal development of the breasts, pubic hair, genitals, and other female sexual characteristics, but women who have pure Turner's syndrome do not ovulate and are thus completely sterile. Adoption and surrogacy are the best choices for these women.

Pregnancy is possible for women with one form of Turner's syndrome, but there are high rates of miscarriages, stillbirths, and chromosomal abnormalities like Down's syndrome in babies conceived by these women. Talk with a genetics counselor and an infertility specialist to help you decide what course of action is best for you.

There are other very rare congenital ovarian disorders whose causes are primarily unknown. These include resistant ovary syndrome, premature ovarian failure, and gonadal agenesis. In some instances, viral and metabolic influences are suspected as causes during the early pregnancy of the mother. Some conditions may be temporary and respond to fertility drugs. Discuss options with your infertility specialist.

BENIGN POLYCYSTIC OVARIAN DISEASE

Benign polycystic ovarian disease, or Stein-Leventhal syndrome, is a common problem in women under thirty. The ovaries develop tiny benign cysts and a thick encapsulating shell when the follicles, which normally burst to release an egg during ovulation, fail to erupt but continue to grow just under the ovarian surface. The syndrome may be caused by a misfunction of the hypothalamus and pituitary or an imbalance between the hormones produced in the ovaries themselves and the adrenal glands. Symptoms can include enlarged painful ovaries, irregular menstruation, infertility, abnormal hair growth, and excessive weight gain.

Infertility caused by polycystic disease frequently responds to Clomid, which increases ovulation. If hormone therapy fails, surgery may be recommended to remove a slice of the ovaries themselves, reducing both the ovarian mass as well as the capsule surrounding it. You should only consider surgery after you have tried other means.

OVARIAN TUMORS

Most ovarian tumors are not malignant, but any enlargement of the ovaries should be thoroughly investigated. A biopsy is usually required for accurate diagnosis of any persistent tumor. (An enlarged ovary does not automatically mean there's a tumor.)

Follicle cysts, which differ from ovarian tumors, can form within a functioning ovary when that follicle does not release its ovum but rather continues to swell and fill with fluid. Individual corpus luteum cysts can also develop. Under normal circumstances after the ovum is released, the corpus luteum naturally disintegrates if pregnancy does not occur. But sometimes the follicle swells and fills with fluid, or with blood (corpus luteum hematoma). When these conditions are corrected, any impaired fertility that you have experienced usually disappears. Benign ovarian cysts often dissipate by themselves.

Ovarian tumors usually do not produce any symptoms, but some women may feel pain during intercourse, and, in time, a sensation of pressure or fullness as the tumor grows. Bladder and bowel irregularities may result from pressure to those organs, and blocked blood vessels and lymph nodes can cause varicose veins, hemorrhoids, and swelling of the legs and vulva. If a tumor is large enough, the uterus may even be displaced.

Ovarian tumors can impair fertility by disrupting the menstrual cycle. Some kinds of tumors produce abnormal amounts of either female or male hormones that throw the body all out of whack. "Feminizing" tumors can mimic pregnancy and can also cause very early puberty in young girls, irregular periods, and abnormal bleeding. Often the endometrial lining and uterus grow abnormally large. Much less frequent are "masculinizing" tumors that can cause menstruation to stop, facial and chest hair to grow, the voice to deepen, and the female body to lose its rounded contours, including a decrease in breast size and an increase in the size of the clitoris. Removing such tumors reverses these changes and the symptoms disappear.

The prognosis for a malignant ovarian tumor depends on the tissue type and stage at which it was detected. Often such tumors aren't discovered until the cancer is advanced. Chemotherapy drugs may render some women infertile or subfertile. And under some circumstances, oncologists will recommend against trying to become pregnant since the heightened hormonal activity of pregnancy may increase the chances for cancer recurrence. But it is also true that pregnancy may be possible, depending on the type of treatment received, and not all oncologists will recommend against it. Carefully question your health-care providers.

Persistent or large ovarian tumors require surgery. Your doctor will undoubtedly try to save your ovaries if you hope to have children. Always discuss this in advance. If one ovary has been removed, pregnancy is still possible if the remaining ovary is functioning. Many women assume that they are only "half as fertile" in such a situation, but this is not so. The remaining ovary will ovulate each month during the regular menstrual cycle.

AN IMPORTANT THING YOU CAN DO

If you have had ovarian surgery, give yourself enough time to heal—at least three months—before attempting to become pregnant.

#8

LEARN HOW TO RECOGNIZE CORPUS LUTEUM PROBLEMS

The corpus luteum is the remains of the burst follicle that encased the egg before it was released. After ovulation, the corpus luteum continues to produce progesterone. Normally, if you have not become pregnant eight to ten days after ovulation, the corpus luteum begins to deteriorate.

But in some women, the deterioration begins after only four or five days, making the last half of the menstrual cycle unusually short. This is called luteal insufficiency, and the normal amounts of progesterone and estrogen are not produced during the menstrual cycle. The lining of the endometrium is therefore inadequate, and a fertilized egg cannot successfully implant there.

Recurrent miscarriages can result from such luteal insufficiency because the corpus luteum is vital during the first three months of pregnancy. During this time, the corpus luteum continues to grow and produce the high levels of hormones necessary to enrich the endometrium encompassing the embryo.

Infertility due to luteal insufficiency results not from

trouble with fertilization but from an inability to maintain the pregnancy at its earliest stages. Vaginal suppositories containing progesterone used during the last half of the menstrual cycle and during the first three months of pregnancy have been successful in helping correct the deficiency. Low doses of HCG and Clomid have also been successfully used to help maintain the corpus luteum. But you should avoid the use of synthetic progestogens like medroxyprogesterone or norethindrone in early pregnancy, because they may damage the fetus.

AN IMPORTANT THING YOU CAN DO

Take your medication at the same time every day to insure that your bloodstream maintains the right hormone levels.

#9

RESEARCH FALLOPIAN
TUBE DISORDERS

The fallopian tubes are small muscular conduits that connect the ovaries to the uterus. After ovulation, the fringed end of the fallopian tube (fimbria) must catch the egg and then gradually pass it along to the ampulla, a wider section in the tube lined with secretory cells, where it can be fertilized by sperm. After fertilization, the egg must be moved through the rest of the tube at exactly the right time to reach the uterus for implantation.

Like the intestines, the fallopian tubes are muscular organs; therefore, their motility—or ability to spontaneously contract and relax—is vital to their successful function. Anything that damages fallopian motility can impair fertility, including any scarring or blockage of the tubes themselves or of the fimbriated end of the tube that must initially pick up the egg.

Tubal blockages and scars can be caused by pelvic inflammatory disease (PID). Pelvic infections affect close to one million American women per year and can occur after abortions and deliveries, from IUDs, gonorrhea, chlamydia, and a wide variety of other organisms. Infertility resulting from damaged tubes affects one in eight women after a single episode of PID, and increases to an alarming 75 percent of women after three or more episodes. A ruptured appendix can also spread infection to the reproductive organs.

Tubal damage and blockage are also caused by endometriosis, a condition in which the endometrial lining grows outside of the uterine region. Tubal damage is also the major cause of ectopic pregnancy, in which a fertilized egg implants in the tube instead of traveling to the uterus. A tubal pregnancy can be life-threatening as well as a cause of infertility.

Sometimes tubal blockage is intentional; for example, women can choose to have their tubes "tied" (tubal ligation) as a means of birth control. In many cases, it is surgically possible to reverse this procedure in order to have children.

Sometimes tubal damage is too extensive to repair surgically, but often damaged sections can be cut away and the ends can be rejoined to create functioning fallopian tubes. This is major surgery using microscopic devices to illuminate the tiny blood vessels and tissues of the tubes. The success or failure of the procedure will depend on the skill of the surgeon and on the position and the amount of blockage that needs to be removed.

AN IMPORTANT THING YOU CAN DO

If you have a reproductive history that includes any of the problems listed above and are actively trying to become pregnant, it is important to be examined and tested for broad-spectrum venereal infections (many of which can exist without symptoms), especially if you have been unable to conceive.

#10

INVESTIGATE UTERINE DISORDERS

In order for the fertilized egg to implant in the uterus, where it will grow and thrive and become a new life, the uterus has to be in good shape, both physically and hormonally. Dysfunctions of the estrogen/progesterone interplay can hinder the proper growth of the endometrial lining and affect implantation. Sometimes the fertilized egg arrives too soon or too late and the endometrium is not ready.

Uterine scars also can create infertility. Scar tissue can form from past injury due to venereal infection, trouble with an IUD, tuberculosis, poor abortion techniques, or a too-diligent dilation and curettage (D & C). This scar tissue can make the endometrial lining rough and impede normal, even blood flow.

On occasion, a thin web of scar tissue can form over the opening between the uterus and fallopian tube. This is an obscure cause of infertility that will only show up during a hysteroscopy, a procedure that uses a direct-viewing tube inserted through the cervix into the uterus. Three to five percent of hysteroscopies reveal such webbing, which can trap and block sperm or stop a fertilized egg from reaching the uterus. Such webbing can usually be removed through the hysteroscope during the procedure.

Sometimes the endometrial lining becomes infected. This disorder, called endometritis, can result from sexually transmitted diseases, but sometimes it may have no apparent cause. If antibiotics do not clear up the infection, a D & C may be recommended to scrape away the infected endometrial tissue.

Nonmalignant fibroid tumors can disrupt the uterus, making implantation a problem. The uterine cavity itself can also be distorted by a congenital abnormality that creates either a "double" uterus or a dividing wall within the uterus called a septum. Such disorders generally cause repeated miscarriages or premature delivery. Do not confuse fibroid tumors with uterine polyps, which are often small and can be removed by a D & C.

Unsuccessful implantation due to infection is usually successfully treated with antibiotics. A septum can be surgically removed. A double uterus, which is often heart-shaped, requires major surgical reconstruction.

Dealing with fibroid tumors is complex. The surgical removal of fibroids, called myomectomy, leaves the uterus intact. Some doctors consider this only a temporary measure, since as many as 20 percent of women with this condition will later require a hysterectomy (removal of the entire uterus). But myomectomy can give women who want children the time they need to become pregnant.

Women who have had a myomectomy and then become pregnant will probably have to deliver by cesarean section, since the myomectomy causes scar tissue in the uterus, which sometimes prevents safe vaginal birth. Myomectomy is more difficult technically than hysterectomy and can cause more blood loss. It is not recommended if the fibroids are large and the uterus is very distorted by their growth. Consult an infertility specialist.

AN IMPORTANT THING YOU CAN DO

If you have had uterine surgery, it is possible that when you become pregnant, a cesarean delivery will be recommended. Get some books and read up on what to expect from such a procedure. Talk with your doctor about it well in advance.

#11

GET TO KNOW YOUR CERVICAL MUCUS

The cervix is like a door to the uterus, and the mucus around it at different times in the menstrual cycle can either open or close the passageway. If the mucus is too thick, sperm cannot penetrate it and infertility results. A chemical pH that is too acidic can be toxic to sperm. Both of these conditions can be caused by hormonal imbalances.

Other cervical mucus problems can result from chronic low-grade infections or inflammation that can cause white blood cells to permeate the cervical mucus, blocking the sperm. Cervicitis is inflammation of the cervical glands and is not uncommon in women who have just given birth. Usually, it clears up by itself without treatment. In other cases, cervicitis is accompanied by a profuse whitish discharge. Women sometimes develop immunological responses to their partner's sperm and produce antibodies to the sperm in the cervical area.

Either systemic or localized antibiotics can be used to treat infections that cause cervical mucus problems. Cervical inflammation will often clear up without treatment. If the condition becomes chronic, however, there are several painless surgical procedures available. Cryosurgery (freezing) or the application of silver nitrate to the cervical area will restructure the surface skin layers, cauterizing the glands and making the cervix smoother when it heals and therefore less prone to infection. This should be done only as a last resort, since there is a possibility that too much mucus-producing tissue can be destroyed.

Infertility due to thick mucus can be caused by too much progesterone or too little estrogen. Estrogen therapy at midcycle often alleviates the difficulty by thinning the mucus and creating the proper alkaline pH balance to accommodate sperm.

AN IMPORTANT THING YOU CAN DO

Pay attention to cervical mucus at different points in your menstrual cycle. Notice any changes in consistency, color, or amount and write them down for your doctor.

#12

Do Not Despair About Past Miscarriages

An inability to carry a pregnancy to term is also a form of infertility. Upwards of 80 percent of women who experience habitual miscarriages eventually carry babies to term in normal pregnancies, so if this has happened to you, do not despair.

Approximately 10 to 15 percent of all confirmed pregnancies end in a miscarriage (spontaneous abortion), usually during the first trimester. An estimated 20 percent of all implanted ova will abort and 50 to 60 percent of all fertilized eggs never progress to a chemically identified pregnancy. Infertility due to miscarriage is sometimes considered a misnomer because the difficulty is not in conceiving but in maintaining the pregnancy.

Many things can cause a woman to abort spontaneously; in fact, early miscarriage is so common that physicians usually do not become alarmed for their patients until they've miscarried three times. It is not at all unusual for women to lose two pregnancies in a row, especially during the first trimester.

Many early pregnancies are lost without the woman even knowing she was pregnant.

Until the mid 1960s, women were considered "habitual aborters" if they had three miscarriages. The definition was thought to include an 80 to 90 percent chance of experiencing another abortion, but we now know that the risks are much lower—around 25 to 30 percent despite the number of previous miscarriages.

There is a slightly higher rate of increased miscarriage among women who have no living children or have had at least one stillbirth or early neonatal death, and in women over age thirty-five. Some of the things that can cause miscarriages are:

- Genetic abnormalities in the fetus
- Chronic maternal illness, such as diabetes, thyroid disorders, heart and kidney problems, and immune system disorders such as systemic lupus erythematosus
- Maternal infections and viruses
- Uterine and cervical disorders
- Corpus luteum and hormonal disorders
- Exposure to environmental and workplace toxins
- Immunologic factors

GENETIC ABNORMALITIES IN THE FETUS

At least 50 to 60 percent of miscarriages in the first trimester are due to known chromosomal abnormalities, many of which are incompatible with life and simply are not found in living babies. The frequency of such abnormalities may be much higher than this since many women miscarry without knowing that they're pregnant. If you have experienced three miscarriages, genetic counseling is probably in order for both partners.

MATERNAL INFECTIONS AND VIRUSES

Some maternal infections and viruses may lead to habitual miscarriage; others can cause single episodes of miscarriage or birth defects in children carried to term.

Bacteria and viruses can affect the fetus by either crossing the placenta through the mother's circulation (the mother may or may not be ill) or by ascending from the vagina through the cervix into the uterus and fetal membranes.

Infections may exist at the time of conception or be contracted shortly into the pregnancy. Most viral infections cause congenital defects by involving the fetal central nervous system, and the earlier in the pregnancy this occurs, the more damaging the result, since this is the most sensitive time for formation of the major fetal organs. Infections that may cause habitual miscarriage include the following:

- Chlamydia, ureaplasma, and mycoplasma: these infections are caused by microbes placed somewhere between bacteria and viruses, and constitute a relatively new category of infections about which much is being learned. They are sexually transmitted diseases believed to be some of the most rampant today. Tetracycline is used to treat both partners (erythromycin is used to treat pregnant women). They can be asymptomatic and may cause repeated miscarriages.
- Herpes virus: Genital herpes infections during the early months of pregnancy can cause miscarriage. Herpes is also sexually transmitted.

Some infections that can cause a single miscarriage include rubella, measles, mumps, influenza, and toxoplasmosis.

UTERINE AND CERVICAL DISORDERS

A misshapen uterus, benign fibroid tumors or polyps, and membrane walls (septa) in the uterus can cause repeated miscarriages. With corrective surgery, the chances are very good for a successful pregnancy. Miscarriages due to these problems tend to occur during the second or third trimester.

Sometimes uterine adhesions, or bands of scar tissue, form due to past IUD use, infections, or too-rough D & C procedures. These adhesions can cause implantation problems and miscarriage. Laser and microsurgery can remove them and improve your chances for a successful pregnancy.

Cervical disorders can also cause miscarriage. *Incompetent cervix* is the term used to describe the premature, progressive relaxation of the cervical tissue that allows the cervix to open and results in lost pregnancy. There is no labor, just the literal feeling of "losing everything." The cause is not completely known but the condition is more common in women with histories of incompetent cervix, in those who have had multiple induced abortions and gynecological procedures such as cervical conization or cauterization, and in those whose mothers used DES during pregnancy. Pregnancy loss due to incompetent cervix usually occurs during the fourth to sixth month of gestation.

Weekly examinations beginning around the twelfth week are recommended for any woman who has lost two second-trimester pregnancies to see if the cervix is opening prematurely. If detected in time, it is possible to stitch the cervix closed (cerclage) under anesthesia to allow the pregnancy to continue to term.

Although not foolproof, cerclage has helped many women bear children they would have lost otherwise. Such preventive measures are sometimes recommended to women with a history of incompetent cervix long before the problem begins. Many doctors suggest preventive stitching around the fourteenth week and, while still controversial, some even recommend it prior to becoming pregnant in women with such a history. The stitch is removed when labor begins.

CORPUS LUTEUM AND HORMONAL DISORDERS

The corpus luteum deteriorates if pregnancy does not occur. But when you become pregnant, the corpus luteum kicks into a high hormone-producing phase to enrich the endometrium that safely encompasses and nourishes the embryo. So great is this production that it is not at all uncommon for the ovary to enlarge and become cystic during the first few months of pregnancy. This condition generally reverses itself by the fourth month.

The corpus luteum produces the estrogen and progesterone necessary to sustain your pregnancy during the first months until the placenta takes over this function. Scientists believe that human chorionic gonadotropin (HCG) is the hormone that sustains the corpus luteum throughout this period.

Maintaining the proper hormone supply is critical to carrying a pregnancy to term. If a woman has previously miscarried due to hormonal deficiencies, progesterone suppositories, Clomid, and low-dose HCG have proved successful in helping maintain corpus luteum production during the early months. However, you should avoid synthetic progestogens during the first months of pregnancy because they may damage the fetus. Ask your doctor about this. You will need to change medication before pregnancy begins if you are taking synthetic progestogens.

EXPOSURE TO ENVIRONMENTAL AND WORKPLACE TOXINS

Studies have shown that women who work in operating rooms and are exposed to anesthetic gases have an increased rate of miscarriage. There is also an increased incidence of miscarriage and infertility among women and men who work in paint manufacturing and plastics industries that use industrial solvents. There have been infrequent reports of "clusters" of miscarriages among office workers who use cathode ray tube (CRT) computer terminals.

Women who work in the metallurgy, electronics, and radio and television manufacturing industries also have higher miscarriage rates. Metallurgy increases exposures to lead, arsenic, cadmium, copper, and mercury. Electronics increases exposure to acid solvent baths. Radio and television manufacturing increases exposure to soldering fumes.

Beauticians and cosmetologists are also exposed to chemicals in hair dyes, permanents, and sprays known to cause miscarriages. Some textile workers may be affected by toxic dust particles from synthetic fabrics.

Immunologic Factors

Thirty percent of women who repeatedly miscarry do not have a genetic, endocrine, gynecologic, or bacterial reason for doing so. These women may have a specific immunologic reaction to their partner's sperm. Women with antisperm antibodies have a 50 percent miscarriage rate. And it is possible that bacterial infections may be present that stimulate the body to produce antibodies that then interpret sperm as "foreign."

To combat this problem, some women can be injected with white blood cells (lymphocytes) taken from their partners. These injections are usually repeated at six-week intervals, and can make some women whose bodies reject their partner's sperm good candidates for successful pregnancies.

AN IMPORTANT THING YOU CAN DO

Since habitual miscarriage can be caused by so many things, it's important to find out what's causing it in you. Be tested for a broad range of infections. Don't despair. Many of the causes are treatable. It will also help to know the early warning signs of miscarriage. Some miscarriages can be averted if you seek help immediately.

#13

UNDERSTAND HOW FEMALE SEXUAL DYSFUNCTION AFFECTS FERTILITY

Although sexual dysfunction is more commonly a cause of male infertility (as discussed in #24), sometimes anxiety-related forms can lead to infertility in women as well. Women sooner lose the desire for sex, as opposed to the actual ability to "perform" the way men do. It is for this reason that only those aspects of female sexual dysfunction that impair fertility are discussed here. (For example, the inability to have an orgasm, though considered a female sexual dysfunction, does not impair a woman's ability to have a child.)

VAGINISMUS

Some women suffer from vaginismus, a sudden, involuntary, spastic reflex of the vaginal muscles that makes penetration impossible. The muscle contractions can occur anytime during the sexual response cycle, either at the beginning of stimulation or when the woman thinks her partner is about to attempt penetration. Vaginismus sometimes arises from anxiety associated with painful sexual episodes, such as incest, rape, or other sexual situations in which a woman felt violated or shamed.

Gradually sized vaginal dilators that the woman inserts herself over a period of time have been found to help. Including her partner in this, using both her fingers and his, often helps ease sexual tension and can resensitize the vagina to pleasurable sensations.

PHOBIC AVOIDANCE OF SEX

Vaginismus can accompany a phobic avoidance of sex, another form of female sexual dysfunction that occurs even in women who ardently want to become pregnant. Some women may express full panic phobias sexually; others may express culturally derived antisexual attitudes in terms of sexual conflict. Distinguishing between the two will help determine a course of treatment since panic disorders, unlike antisexual attitudes, may respond to certain medications.

It is important to keep in mind that sexual relations, pregnancy, and intimacy can panic either spouse and that proper professional and personal attention should help alleviate it.

AN IMPORTANT THING YOU CAN DO

Find a therapist skilled in women's sexual difficulties. It's important to get to the root causes. A sympathetic therapist whom you trust can help a great deal.

PART THREE

MALE INFERTILITY

#14

KNOW WHAT CAUSES
INFERTILITY IN MEN

If you are having difficulty conceiving, many potential causes can be easily eliminated by testing the male partner first. Causes of male infertility are often more easily diagnosed than those of female infertility, because sperm samples are more readily obtained for analysis than, for example, information about fallopian tube motility.

For several years, researchers have been shocked to find declining sperm counts in men across the United States. Possible causes include exposure to environmental and workplace toxins, many of which are considered "safe," some electromagnetic fields, stress, and substance abuse.

Knowledge of male infertility is light-years behind what is already known about women's infertility. That's because up until the 1950s, men were considered fertile if they were capable of getting an erection and producing even small amounts of sperm. While our understanding of male fertility is more advanced today, more research in this area is needed.

Infertility in men can be relative. Fewer than 2 percent of

infertile men, for example, are completely sterile. But defining the situation for men is much more complex than doing so for women. There is rarely only one cause, and most male fertility problems are a combination of several, sometimes small, factors.

Infertility in men can be caused by:

- Abnormal sperm production due to hormonal imbalances, radiation therapy, genital abnormalities, genetic factors, elevated temperature in the genital region, autoimmunity or antisperm antibodies, medications, and substance abuse
- Blockage of the sperm flow due to sexually transmitted diseases, past surgery, accidents, congenital anomalies, and physiological disorders
- Sexual dysfunction, such as impotence, premature ejaculation, retarded ejaculation, and other ejaculatory disorders
- Illnesses like mumps and diabetes
- Sperm damage due to exposure to environmental toxins and some electromagnetic fields

AN IMPORTANT THING YOU CAN DO

Try not to "awfulize" your situation. Many men with impaired fertility feel "less than a man." Know that infertility is common in men today. You are not alone! And there are many things that can be done to improve fertility.

#15

FIND OUT MORE ABOUT
SPERM PRODUCTION

Men often have vague ideas about sperm production that can
be quite inaccurate. Since knowledge is power, finding out as
much as you can about it can only help.

During ejaculation, a man releases, on average, between
40 and 150 million sperm, about 90 percent of which are killed
off by various vaginal fluids. Men who typically ejaculate less
than 60 million sperm may have difficulty fathering a child,
but sperm count alone is not the most important criterion in
sperm analysis.

The *quality* of the sperm is essential. Defective sperm is
responsible for the vast majority of male infertility problems.
Many men with low sperm counts have fathered children
without difficulty, while some men with high sperm counts
have not. The criteria that determine good sperm quality are
motility—how fast, easily, and straight sperm swims; normal
size, shape, and character; balanced viscosity or stickiness; and
a general fluid volume within normal ranges.

HORMONAL INFLUENCES ON SPERM

Although men do not experience the cyclic hormonal changes that women do in monthly patterns, some of the same basic reproductive hormones are common to both sexes. Men produce millions of sperm daily, which requires the continued presence of FSH and LH generated by the hypothalamus and pituitary glands. Anything that hinders this production or creates imbalance will automatically affect fertility through decreased sperm production.

As in women, fertility in men often reflects overall good health. Brain tumors and infections like encephalitis, as well as small tumors of the hypothalamus and pituitary, can disrupt the functioning of those areas and reduce the production of FSH and LH. This in turn will cause the testicles to atrophy, and since sperm is produced in the testicles, infertility results.

When the hormone imbalance is fixed in women, fertility usually returns. Hormone treatment in men has not shown much promise to date, however. Luckily, infertility in men due to hormonal disturbances is rare and accounts for only about 15 percent of cases seen in infertility clinics. By comparison, 40 percent of female infertility results from hormonal imbalance.

There is much confusion about the actual role, if any, of testosterone in sperm production. Testosterone is the potent hormone present in both men and women that stimulates sex drive. Many people assume that it is responsible for male "virility," which conjures up images of a hairy chest, big muscles, and an accompanying high sperm count. However, this is not the case. Testosterone is responsible for the growth of the sex organs, facial and chest hair, and the deepening of the voice during puberty. But it has little to do with a man's physique, which is determined by heredity.

Sperm production and testosterone are the products of different cell systems. Sperm production is controlled by FSH (in Sertoli cells); testosterone production is controlled by LH (in Leydig cells), within the testicles. The cells that produce

sperm are fragile and easily damaged, but the cells that produce testosterone are rugged and rarely frail. This is why it's
possible for a man to have a low sperm count while maintaining all the signs of sexual potency. "Virile" men with low
sperm counts can find this extremely disturbing.

What's known about the effect of testosterone on sperm
production is that a little is required, but too much will stop it
altogether. That's why the sperm count falls when testosterone supplements are given. The brain, in response to the
extra hormone, thinks the testicles are overproducing it and
cuts down the FSH supply, which in turn does not allow the
testicles to manufacture sperm. In addition, the testicles also
stop making their own supply of testosterone. When the supplements are stopped, normal production levels return.

Sometimes the adrenal glands, which are located on top
of the kidneys and produce the same hormones in both men
and women, can produce excess male hormones. The brain
perceives this increase as if it were coming from the testicles
and the cycle described above ensues.

An excess of thyroid hormone can also reduce fertility in
men. However, this is very rare since symptoms of hyperthyroidism usually warrant medical supervision long before they
affect fertility.

The hormonal system in men rarely falters the way it
does in women, perhaps because of its steady, nonshifting nature. Although male hormones may be altered slightly on a
daily basis due to factors such as stress, fatigue, illness, and
frequency of ejaculation, they do not go through major phases
on a twenty-eight-day cycle with different hormones dominat-
ing at different times. Men produce and maintain consistently
high levels of hormones.

Unfortunately, hormonal treatments for men who have
imbalances are not as developed as those for women. Researchers have reported both positive and negative sperm-
production responses in men who have taken Clomid, and
Pergonal has shown some promise. But the prevailing attitude

is that even though hormonal therapy for men may not hurt, chances are it won't help much either. More study is needed.

AN IMPORTANT THING YOU CAN DO

Talk with your doctor about trying a few courses of fertility drugs to temporarily improve sperm production if your difficulties are hormone-related. Set a time frame beyond which you will stop taking the medication.

#16

PROTECT YOUR SPERM
FROM RADIATION

Since X rays were discovered at the turn of the century, we've known that ionizing radiation damages sperm production by affecting the spermatogonia (mother cells) that create sperm in the testicles without harming the other reproductive support cells. This damage can be severe enough to make fertilization unlikely or to produce chromosomal abnormalities that can cause birth defects. Damaged spermatogonia have the ability to regenerate in time, thereby producing sperm, but birth defects can result if the DNA code has been altered.

Men should always be careful to guard themselves against any X-ray or other ionizing radiation exposures. Men who work in a radiation-related job, such as X-ray technicians, dentists, doctors, and workers in food irradiation or the nuclear industry, must take precautions to shield their testicular area with an appropriate lead apron, as well as wear badges that reflect daily exposures. Any man who goes for X rays of any part of the body should be sure to request a shield for the genital area.

Men who have undergone radiation therapy for genital or testicular tumors should have a sperm analysis done afterward. The dosage of radiation needed to kill malignant cells in an affected testicle is high enough to affect the nonirradiated testicle. Although the healthy testicle would have been shielded during therapy and will continue to produce sperm, it's likely some DNA damage occurred. Talk with your doctor before trying to become a parent.

AN IMPORTANT THING YOU CAN DO

Always protect your genital area when having X rays taken, even if they are dental X rays. See #33 for information on non-ionizing radiation.

#17

LEARN WHICH TESTICULAR
ABNORMALITIES YOU CAN CORRECT

Some men are born with testicular abnormalities that will cause infertility during the reproductive years if left untreated. They are often detected either at birth or in early puberty and are best corrected then. But other genital abnormalities can develop later in life such as varicoceles or torsion (the sudden twisting of a testicle, which is a medical emergency. See #22, p. 70). And sometimes the testicles withdraw into a man's body during lovemaking.

In order for sperm to be made in the testicles, the testicles must function at a temperature slightly lower than normal body temperature. Elevated temperature for any reason decreases sperm production. If the testicles do not descend from the interior abdominal cavity into the scrotal sac, their temperature will be the same as the body's interior temperature, which is too high for sperm production.

Undescended testicles affects one in 200 newborn males. It is usually treated before the age of two with hormone therapy or microsurgery.

At one time, physicians used to wait to see if the testicles would descend on their own during puberty. But today, it's known that to wait that long could permanently impair fertility.

A diagnosis of undescended testicles is usually made at birth. The hormone HCG is administered between age six and eighteen months to raise testosterone levels. If the testicles do not descend in response to this treatment, then microsurgery is recommended as soon as possible. Treatment should be completed by age two.

Sometimes only one testicle will descend. Fertility is still possible, but the remaining testicle will atrophy inside the body, and surgery will be ineffective unless it is performed in the first years.

Sometimes the testicles will withdraw into the body when a man has an erection. Unless intercourse is prolonged, meaning the temperature of the testicles is elevated enough to affect the sperm, fertility should not be impaired.

AN IMPORTANT THING YOU CAN DO

If one or both of your testicles withdraws inside your body during lovemaking, gently press on your lower abdomen to release it.

#18

FIND OUT IF A GENETIC DISORDER IS AFFECTING YOUR FERTILITY

Some genetic disorders can impair a man's fertility. Here are some of the better-known ones.

KALLMAN'S SYNDROME

Kallman's syndrome, a disorder of the hypothalamus that retards its ability to release LH-RH, is probably genetically based but no one is sure. What is known is that the central nervous system doesn't develop normally in the embryo. Men with Kallman's typically do not finish development of puberty, and are tall and skinny. Other common characteristics include very soft testicles, no sense of smell, color blindness, deafness, and cleft lip and palate. These characteristics vary greatly from individual to individual.

A man with Kallman's has no sperm in his ejaculate and all of his hormone levels are low. The treatment that shows the most promise is the administration of LH-RH. Preliminary studies show that men who receive LH-RH may experience full sexual maturation with normal sperm production. Pergonal is also used effectively. The earlier the diagnosis is made, the better the chances are for successful treatment.

Klinefelter's Syndrome

A man with Klinefelter's syndrome has at least one extra X chromosome, and sometimes more. One to 2 percent of all infertile men have this disorder. While all chromosomally caused disorders are rare, this is the most common, occurring in 1 in 800 male births.

Most men with Klinefelter's are not aware of it. Physical manifestations are considered within the normal range of masculine appearance. Sometimes it will be noticed during puberty when the testicles do not mature completely. But often, the testicles are just small, breasts very slightly enlarged, and there is a slight feminine appearance. It is usually infertility that brings a man to treatment.

Unfortunately, nothing can be done to reverse the XXY chromosome pattern, and men with this disorder will be permanently infertile. Sex drive may be diminished due to a decrease in testosterone production. Additional testosterone may increase sex drive.

In some instances, those with Klinefelter's express it in what's called a mosaic pattern, meaning some cells carry XXY information while others carry a normal XY combination. In such cases, it may be possible, with hormone therapy, to produce some sperm, thereby allowing the possibility for children.

Sertoli-Cell-Only Syndrome

In very rare cases, spermatogonia (mother cells that generate sperm) are missing altogether, probably since birth. Tests usually reveal that everything else, with the exception of very slightly elevated hormone levels, is normal, yet there is no sperm. The cause is unknown but genetics may be a fac-

tor. There is no treatment for this disorder. Men with Sertoli-
Cell-Only syndrome find their best chances of fatherhood are
in artificial insemination using a donor's sperm or adoption.

AN IMPORTANT THING YOU CAN DO

If no cause for your infertility can be found, consider having a
blood test for genetic problems. Depending on the results, try
a few courses of hormone therapy.

19

Keep Your Genital Temperature Cool

It's important that a man's genital temperature be cooler than average body temperature in order for normal sperm production to occur. Another factor (besides undescended testicles) which decreases sperm production through elevated temperature is a twisted or enlarged varicose vein within the testicle called a varicocele. A varicocele increases blood circulation and can impair fertility by elevating temperature.

Between 30 and 40 percent of infertile men will be found to have a varicocele. It is among the most common causes of male infertility and is also the most treatable today.

A varicocele can be tied off in surgery under local or general anesthesia. Sperm production typically improves after this procedure, resulting in a 50 percent successful pregnancy rate. Before opting for surgery, many men try alternatives such as wearing testicular cooling devices and hormone treatments. The alternatives show a 30 percent success rate.

Some kinds of employment can raise testicular temperature. Truck drivers, for instance, sit on very warm seats for many hours during the day, which theoretically would reduce the sperm count. The CB radios in their cabs (positioned within arm's reach at the genital level) operate in the FM frequency band known to heat tissue. Men who work around AM/FM radio and television broadcast towers, cellular phone transmitters, or radar equipment, including handheld radar guns in police patrol cars, can also experience decreased sperm counts. (See #33, p. 109.) Working in occupations where temperatures reach 120 degrees Fahrenheit, such as welding or boiler maintenance or operation, can also suppress sperm production. Levels usually return to normal when the heat source is removed.

Oxygen deprivation or saturation may also reduce sperm counts. Sperm-producing cells, which need a lot of oxygen to function, shut down when oxygen is diminished. Working at extremes of altitudes (above 5,000 feet or 100 feet below the sea) can therefore suppress sperm production. Men who relocate from sea level to higher altitudes may experience a temporary drop. In divers the drop is probably caused by a saturation of oxygen in the blood's red cells. Sperm reduction in these cases is considered transient.

AN IMPORTANT THING YOU CAN DO

Carefully examine your lifestyle, employment, and hobbies for anything that might elevate genital temperature. Wear loose boxer shorts rather than tight-fitting briefs, which hold the genitals close to the body.

#20

INVESTIGATE AUTOIMMUNITY

One of the more baffling instances of male infertility is when a man develops antibodies to his own sperm. These antibodies circulate in the bloodstream and prevent healthy sperm production in a volume necessary for fertility.

Past infection or injury may be two reasons why this happens. Both of these can cause obstruction in tubal areas, which then cause sperm to spill over into other genital tissue. The body reacts by setting up an immune response, creating antibodies that attack the sperm as if it is foreign.

Treating infertility due to autoimmune responses that kill sperm is difficult and often involves trying to trick the man's body out of perceiving his sperm as an unwanted invader. Reducing sperm production through the administration of testosterone often leads to suppression of the unwanted immune response. When this short-term testosterone therapy is stopped, the immune response hopefully is stopped as well. Some centers treat men with

short-term, high-dose cortisone derivatives that also suppress sperm production.

AN IMPORTANT THING YOU CAN DO

Read up on the side effects of cortisone.

#21

Know the Effects of Medications on Your Fertility

Many medications, including over-the-counter drugs, can have an unexpected impact on male fertility. What's safe to take in "normal" times may tilt the scales in the wrong direction when you are trying to father a child.

A number of medications taken regularly may inhibit sperm production, including large doses of aspirin. Prescription medications known to decrease sperm production include cortisone, which is a synthetic hormone preparation similar to the natural hormone cortisol, which is produced in the adrenal glands; corticosteroids, which are anti-inflammatory drugs prescribed for ailments such as allergies, arthritis, skin disorders, and athletic injuries that have become chronic conditions; and disorders such as systemic lupus erythematosus. Medications for depression and for high blood pressure can also reduce normal hormonal production through their action on the brain.

Chemotherapy, which interferes with DNA replication, can also reduce sperm production. These drugs work by taking the place of certain vitamins during cell synthesis, thereby impairing the system so that the malignant cells die off. Sperm production often returns when chemotherapy is stopped. Researchers continue to look for other drugs, and different applications, that will have less affect on the reproductive system.

AN IMPORTANT THING YOU CAN DO

Talk to your doctor about the possibility of not using some medications while trying to conceive. Be sure to tell your doctor if you take lots of vitamins or use aspirin regularly.

#22

UNDERSTAND WHAT BLOCKS
SPERM FLOW

Sperm travels a considerable distance from its original production site in the testicles to its eventual destination through the urethra into the vagina. The tubes, ducts, and temporary storage areas involved are fragile sites and any obstruction or divergence along the way will cause infertility.

Produced in the testicles, mature sperm is stored within eighteen feet of tightly coiled tube called the epididymis. It must travel through this tube before reaching the vas deferens, the tube that connects the epididymis to the prostate gland area. (The vas deferens is the tube that is sealed during a vasectomy.) The sperm is mixed with fluid from the prostate and other glands, and this mixture, called semen, becomes the ejaculate. Infertility can result from any blockage or misdirection along this path, as well as from poor quality or quantity of the fluid that accompanies the sperm.

Blockage problems cause about 5 percent of male infertility. In a few cases incomplete development of ducts produces blockage disorders, but most blockages occur later in life as a result of injury or infection.

A urological examination—the male equivalent of the gynecological examination—is essential for determining the causes of infertility. Most blockages and their suspected causes can be discovered and a course of treatment recommended, such as antibiotics, anti-inflammatory drugs, and surgery. Microsurgery has come a long way in helping to restore fertility to many men.

Like a woman's fallopian tubes, the tubes that sperm travel through require a certain motility. They are not just hollow passageways; scar tissue can form within them for several reasons, causing a thickening that results in blockage.

PAST INFECTIONS

The most common sources of obstruction are injury, inflammation, and infection. Once these are treated, fertility often returns. Some sexually transmitted diseases, which can be asymptomatic in men, cause scarring. Bacterial infections like gonorrhea and chlamydia (the most frequently sexually transmitted disease in the United States) are the most common causes of duct scarring. Gonorrhea usually produces painful symptoms in men (though not in women) before the infection advances too far, but chlamydia can be asymptomatic in men as well as women.

Other infections like tuberculosis, which is increasing at an alarming rate in the United States and is still prevalent in third-world countries, can affect male reproduction. TB destroys the passageways of the epididymis and can invade the vas deferens. TB of the reproductive system can also be sexually transmitted to women and make them infertile.

Ureaplasma and mycoplasma, organisms linked to urethritis, can sometimes cause obstructions to the ejaculatory ducts. It can also infect the seminal fluid and damage sperm. Not much is known about these organisms and treatments are often ineffective.

Bacterial and viral infections of the prostate gland can alter semen. The prostate gland seems to harbor bacteria that can leak into semen, killing sperm. From the prostate, bacteria can enter all the seminal ducts and cause blockages. Some prostate infections can also be transmitted to women; others alter the semen's composition, causing it to thicken and the sperm to clump together. Although difficult to treat, most prostate infections eventually respond to antibiotics.

Past Surgery

Surgery can also cause blockages, sometimes years later. Surgical procedures to remove hernias or to repair undescended testicles often come extremely close to spermatic cords and ducts. It is very easy to injure the vas deferens or an artery. Damaged arteries can lead to the death of the testicle. The vas deferens can usually be repaired through microsurgery, but there is always the danger of more scarring from any surgery.

Torsion

In rare instances, blockage can be a spontaneous event in which the testicle twists on its own blood supply. This is known as torsion, and is very painful; the testicle swells dramatically. Torsion is considered a medical emergency. If the testicle is not released within six hours, it will die. A urologist unwinds it and sutures it to adjacent tissue in order to stabilize it.

In the past, men who lost a testicle to torsion were told that the remaining one would compensate. Often, however, men who have gone through this are sterile. This is thought to be due to an immune reaction by the body that sends antibodies in response to the twisted testicle but then kills sperm-producing cells in the other testicle as well.

AN IMPORTANT THING YOU CAN DO

Be sure your doctor checks you for a wide range of infections whether you have symptoms or not. Unfortunately if you live in a major city today, a TB test is also a good idea.

#23

CONSIDER VASECTOMY REVERSAL

Men who have chosen vasectomy as a birth control method may want to reverse the procedure. Often this can be accomplished, but it's best to talk with the doctor who performed the original surgery since that person is most familiar with his or her own surgical techniques, as well as your specific history.

Unfortunately, there has been a 50 percent incidence of an autoimmune response to sperm production in men who have had the operation. This can create problems for those who wish to reverse the procedure and father children, and may even account for the relatively low pregnancy success rates (30 percent) following such reversals. The use of steroid medications to suppress the immune system has been effective in reducing antisperm antibodies.

Reversing the original vasectomy, which probably took less than a half hour in a doctor's office, is far more complicated than the initial procedure. It requires general anesthesia in a hospital and takes more than two hours, in addition to a four- or five-day hospital stay. However, some surgeons

recently have been performing the procedures on an outpatient basis with local anesthesia. Laser surgery, which can
connect fragile tissue together without sutures, shows particular promise.

There is a 30 to 35 percent successful pregnancy rate after vasectomy reversals, and 60 to 80 percent of men are able
to produce at least some viable sperm afterward. It is possible
to collect small amounts of sperm over a period of time and
use it in artificial insemination techniques.

AN IMPORTANT THING YOU CAN DO

If you're considering vasectomy reversal, try to locate the surgeon who did the vasectomy. If that person does not perform
reversals, ask what his or her techniques were so you can take
that information to your new surgeon.

#24

Understand How Male Sexual Dysfunction Affects Fertility

We often automatically assume that sexual dysfunction in men refers only to an inability to get or sustain an erection. But this is not the case. Sperm must be deposited high in the vagina, close to the cervix, in order for fertilization to occur. Anything that restricts this process may impair optimum fertility, including sexual positions that interfere with full penetration, impotence or premature ejaculation, no ejaculation, or retrograde ejaculation into the bladder.

Injuries, discomfort, or simple personal preference may cause couples to adopt sexual positions that restrict full penetration. This is why an infertility counseling session will include questions about sexual positions. Believe it or not, some infertility problems are solved this easily. Others unfortunately are not. But some cases of infertility that are due to sexual dysfunction—such as in paraplegia—are yielding to "high-tech" approaches, allowing men to father children who just a few years ago would not have been able to do so.

HYPOSPADIAS

Hypospadias is a congenital anomaly in which the urethral opening on the penis is found on its underside, at varying distances from the tip, instead of in its normal position at the head of the tip. As a result, ejaculate can be deposited too low in the vagina to reach the cervix in numbers adequate enough for fertilization. Artificial insemination using the father's sperm is a possible solution, however, since the problem is basically one of sperm transport.

PREMATURE EJACULATION

Unfortunately, premature ejaculation is often the brunt of jokes that tap an apparently large reserve of masculine insecurity about the duration of erections. But true premature ejaculation is serious, perplexing, and emotionally painful, and leads to infertility, because fertilization cannot happen unless sperm reaches the top of the vagina.

Not to be confused with simply "coming fast," premature ejaculation involves a near-complete absence of control over the time when ejaculation occurs. A man may ejaculate even before entering his partner's vagina, or, once there, he may ejaculate so quickly that the sperm is not deposited high enough. Often the slightest genital touching brings about ejaculation, which is especially frustrating if a couple is used to ending sexual stimulation with male ejaculation. This problem can lead to impotence, as well as a total lack of sexual desire.

Premature ejaculation is the most common of the male sexual dysfunctions and the most easily treated. It is due more to the inability to recognize the various sensate phases leading to ejaculation than to a lack of "manly control." Learning to recognize these various phases often establishes the ability to control the process by recognizing when to stop stimulation.

It takes time, willingness, emotional openness, and acceptance on the part of both partners to address premature ejaculation in constructive ways, without the blame, recrimination, and watchful judging that sex therapists call "spectatoring." Spectatoring your sensuality can undermine sexual communication, which, in turn, can undermine your relationship in other ways.

Men who suffer from either nonorganic impotence or premature ejaculation benefit greatly by simply learning to identify how anxiety affects them sexually. Learn about your own sexual response, what pleases or does not please both you and your partner. It can be an exciting journey if approached in gentle, nonjudgmental ways. (See the exercises in #46.)

Keep in mind that we all go through phases when we are more or less interested in sex. Lack of interest is natural in physically and emotionally stressful situations such as illness or mourning. There is no reason to worry unless it continues over a protracted period of time.

There are obviously situations in which a lack of sexual desire is a by-product of other things that are happening in your relationship. Attention to them first will often restore sexual interest. Sometimes all it takes is a new environment or an "overnight getaway."

Retarded Ejaculation

The opposite of premature ejaculation is retarded ejaculation, which involves a prolonged erection. When ejaculation finally occurs, it is perceived as unsatisfactory for both partners. Sometimes ejaculation does not happen at all, and people often give up, frustrated, in the middle of lovemaking, when continuing would make both partners feel brutalized. Men invariably become caught up in striving, and women are left feeling inadequate. Sometimes men can ejaculate only during masturbation.

The sensate-focusing exercises discussed in #46 will help to relieve sexual anxiety and striving. Once anxiety is reduced, a man may feel open enough to show his mate the

methods he uses during masturbation. After establishing fa-
miliarity with Sensate Exercises 1 and 2, a man should avoid
penetrating his partner in Sensate Exercise 3 until he senses
ejaculation is near (see #46, pages 157–160).

RETROGRADE EJACULATION

Sometimes a neurologically based disorder will cause a
man to ejaculate back into his bladder rather than out through
the urethra. A normal orgasm is experienced, but there is no
ejaculate. The next urination, however, will be milky white
and filled with semen. The difficulty is usually traced to
weakened nerves that control muscles at the base of the bladder, which normally close off during ejaculation.

Men taking medication for hypertension or depression
can also experience retrograde ejaculation as a side effect,
because these medications weaken the sympathetic nervous
system. It is sometimes the first symptom of sexual dysfunction associated with diabetes. Damage to these nerves
caused by past surgery can sometimes be reversed by corrective surgery.

Although there is no physical danger from retrograde
ejaculation, couples need to solve the problem in order
to conceive.

If your medication is causing retrograde ejaculation, talk
with your doctor about making changes. Diabetic men can
be given medication to stimulate the sympathetic nervous
system into restoring nerve function and reversing retrograde ejaculation.

If medical treatments fail, consider sperm retrieval for artificial insemination. This procedure involves several steps.
The woman must know how to gauge her approaching ovulation. The man is asked to drink one teaspoon of sodium bicarbonate dissolved in a glass of water four times a day for two
days prior to his partner's ovulation. (Sodium bicarbonate neu-
tralizes his urine, which is too acidic for sperm survival.) On

the insemination day, the man is asked to empty his bladder and then masturbate. A urologist inserts a sterile catheter through the penis and retrieves the sperm from the bladder, which is then treated for artificial insemination.

In another approach to retrieving sperm, the man's bladder is washed with a sterile solution hospitable to sperm. The man is then asked to masturbate and urinate immediately into a sterile glass vessel.

IMPOTENCE

Sexual dysfunction problems account for only approximately 5 percent of male infertility, but their psychological impact can be destructive to any intimate relationship, with or without children. When a couple wants children, however, impotence can destroy even the strongest relationship.

Impotence, the inability to get or sustain an erection, obviously leads to infertility. Its causes can be either physical or psychological, or a combination of the two. The percentages are divided about equally among them.

Virtually every man experiences impotence at some time in his life. Occasional episodes are nothing to worry about. Tiredness, worry, alcohol, and just plain bad mood can contribute to temporary impotence. Unfortunately, impotence often terrifies men into a mental state that compounds the problem.

Thirty percent of impotence cases are caused by physical disorders. Prostate and other kinds of surgery, including radical procedures for colorectal cancer, can cause impotence, as well as illnesses like diabetes and endocrine and neurological disorders.

Habitual use of narcotics and alcohol, as well as tranquilizers in the phenothiazine family, can cause impotence, as can some medications for high blood pressure and depression.

If you experience any sudden, or gradual but definite, change in your ability to get an erection, a thorough physical

examination is in order. Serious illness may be behind it. Do
not wait.

Often the cause of impotence lies within the emotional
realm and is quite easy to fall into, kicking off a cycle of performance anxiety, failure to accomplish goals, self-blame, self-
loathing, and shame, until abandoning sex altogether seems to
be the only safe thing to do.

American culture places great emphasis on "performance"
and achieving goals, particularly for men. It also flaunts sex in
the sale of everything from dog food to automobiles. Yet our
deep Puritanical roots often prevent us from developing a mature sense of loving eroticism, denying the legitimate role of relaxed "pleasuring" rather than merely accomplishing orgasms
and pregnancy.

From a strictly physiological standpoint, sexual anxiety
will generally express itself as a lack of desire in women and as
a lack of ability in men. The factors involved can become in-
credibly complex and should be explored with a therapist
trained in the field. Some simple mutual "pleasuring" exercises, aimed at removing "performance pressure" are discussed in #46.

PARAPLEGIA

A tremendous amount has been learned within the last
several decades about spinal cord injuries. Men with such injuries, once considered incapable of fathering children, may
now be able to do so in some instances. But even with today's
advances, less than 10 percent of men with paraplegia will be
able to become fathers. Spinal cord injuries can affect not only
a man's ability to get erections and to ejaculate, but sperm
production can be impaired as well.

The completeness and location of the spinal injury is
often what determines the degree of impotence a man may experience. Partial lesions often do not completely impair potency.

Those with completely severed spinal cords may have more difficulties. There is also a better chance for getting erections when the injury is closer to the neck than the lower back, although the erections may not be strong. The lower the injury on the body, however, the more likely are ejaculation possibilities.

While these basic impaired sexual functions can be understood from a neurological point of view, the damage to sperm quality itself in paraplegics is less well understood. Unfortunately semen quality is poor and sperm often abnormal, probably due to decreased activity in the testicles.

Spinal cord injuries create a three-pronged obstacle to fertility: reduced sperm production, as well as erection and ejaculation difficulties. Erection difficulties can be helped with penile prosthesis implants, while reduced sperm production varies at different times and with different circumstances. The most difficult problem to surmount is an inability to ejaculate.

Two approaches have been tried. One, called electroejaculation, uses low-level electrical stimulation to the rectal and genital area. Semen is then gathered and used for artificial insemination. Several successful pregnancies have resulted from this approach.

The other is more risky. Called chemical ejaculation, it uses intravenous or spinal injections of neostigmine which elevates blood pressure. Done in an intensive care hospital setting with strict monitoring, there are serious risks associated with treatment, including raising the blood pressure to dangerous levels. (Anyone with a history of strokes or cardiovascular disease will not be considered for this.) Artificial insemination of your spouse then follows.

Erections have occurred in approximately 60 percent of chemical ejaculation procedures. Sometimes ejaculation occurs without an erection, and it may spill into the bladder, from which it can be retrieved. But several successful pregnancies have resulted from this technique.

AN IMPORTANT THING YOU CAN DO

If you are experiencing any of the sexual problems described, it's important to seek appropriate help, both medical and psychological. Ask your doctor for a referral to a therapist who specializes in male sexual difficulties. Screen potential therapists carefully to insure that they have the special training necessary for this type of counseling.

#25

UNDERSTAND HOW PREEXISTING
ILLNESSES AFFECT FERTILITY

Any major illness in men that raises body temperature for a prolonged period can cause sperm damage. Usually when body temperature returns to normal, sperm production will, too. Certain illnesses such as diabetes, mumps, nephritis (inflammation of the kidneys), and meningitis may permanently injure the sperm-producing tissues, resulting in irreversible infertility.

DIABETES

Aside from damage to sperm production, diabetes can be quite destructive to a man's sexuality. Progressive damage to tiny blood vessels that destroys minute nerve endings around the penis eventually causes impotence. Twenty-two to 55 percent of all diabetic men are impotent. Some men regain potency when the disease is under control, but for others, impotence becomes permanent.

Although a diabetic man retains his sex drive and ability

to have an orgasm and to ejaculate, the absence of erection makes impregnation impossible without assistance. If you are diabetic but can masturbate into a glass, the ejaculate can be saved and treated for artificial insemination. New treatments include the use of artificial penile prostheses that are surgically implanted. These can be rigid, semirigid, or inflatable. Diabetics often benefit from psychological counseling as well.

MUMPS

Mumps, a viral infection usually of the neck glands, can cause sterility in men who contract it after puberty if it travels to the testicles. Mumps after age fourteen does not automatically lead to sterility; in about half of all cases, the virus does not reach the testicles and there is no problem. Sometimes it reaches only one testicle and the remaining one can compensate by producing sperm. And even when both testicles are damaged, some tubules can recover with time.

The mumps virus is attracted to cells that are dividing quickly. Before puberty, the reproductive cells are relatively inactive, but during puberty, they begin a high degree of cell division. The mumps virus, living in a medium of rapid division, upon which it thrives, can replicate itself millions of times, causing some cells to explode. This is called mumps orchitis, and it can permanently destroy sperm-producing cells.

The good news is that only 18 percent of mumps cases occur in men during or past puberty and in 70 percent of those cases, the virus infects only one testicle; the other continues to function normally. If mumps infects both testicles, the disease is usually stopped before permanent damage occurs. Often, within a year, the cells regenerate enough to produce sperm. Only 5 percent of men who contract mumps become permanently sterile.

Diagnosis of infertility due to mumps is made through a physical examination, a blood test, and a semen analysis. The testicles may be small, a blood test often high in FSH, which the pituitary gland overproduces in response to low hormone messages from the testicles, and little or no sperm will be present. If there is no sperm, then there is unfortunately no treatment. But if there is some sperm, hormone therapy or fertility drugs can be used to increase sperm production.

AN IMPORTANT THING YOU CAN DO

Examine your medical history to see if any preexisting illness or chronic condition may be affecting your fertility.

#26

INVESTIGATE THE EFFECTS OF ENVIRONMENTAL TOXINS ON MALE FERTILITY

We live in a contaminated world. Toxins specifically known to damage sperm or reduce its production in the testicles include industrial compounds such as polychlorinated biphenyls (PCBs), Agent Orange (dioxin), lead, mercury, cadmium, and other heavy metals. Herbicides and pesticides used in agriculture, landscaping, and some municipal road-crew work are also known to damage sperm. Men who live near landfills, municipal incinerators, or factories that produce or use any of these compounds are at higher risk for sperm damage that can cause infertility or birth defects.

Chemical compounds affect sperm by killing it, rearranging the DNA of its nucleus, or causing the sperm-producing cells to begin abnormal division, which leads to cancer. DNA-damaged sperm may look normal under a microscope but may be either incapable of fertilizing an egg, or, if it does, damaged enough to cause birth defects.

The state of sperm analysis for such DNA damage is not at all sophisticated. If you work in industries like the electronics industry, which many consider "clean" but which uses highly toxic solvent baths for circuit boards, you are at risk, and present diagnostic technology cannot assure the safe quality of your sperm.

AN IMPORTANT THING YOU CAN DO

The best course of action is to know what you are working with. Call your state department of environmental protection and ask a lot of questions. Don't stop until you get good answers and don't be easily pacified. If you suspect you are working with hazardous products, in the home as well as on the job, do your best to take precautions or reduce exposure as much as possible. Have your water at work and at home tested by your local health department for chemicals and heavy metals.

#27

RECOGNIZE THAT SOMETIMES IT'S THE INFERTILE "COUPLE"

In the vast majority of cases, infertility can be traced to either one partner or the other. But sometimes the two members of the couple are fertile as individuals yet infertile together.

This situation is extremely perplexing to the people involved and difficult for the medical community to solve. The causes are lodged in the immunology of the conception process, and not much is known about it. The woman's body can reject her partner's sperm at any one of three important points:

1. At the cervix, when an incompatibility exists between her cervical mucus and his sperm
2. In the fallopian tubes, when incompatibility exists during fertilization itself
3. In the uterus, when proper capacitation fails to occur as the sperm passes through

CAPACITATION

Capacitation is not well understood medically but immunologic interactions are suspected. In 1951, during tests on rabbits, scientists found that the sperm, when it entered the vagina, was not automatically capable of fertilizing the egg. Some substance or substances in the uterus or fallopian tubes activates enzymes in the head of the sperm. This process is called capacitation, and it must occur before sperm can penetrate the egg's outer coating. It is clear that for fertility to exist between partners, the physiological interaction between them must be a positive, compatible one.

ADVERSE IMMUNOLOGICAL RESPONSE

For unknown reasons, some women develop antibodies to their partner's sperm. The body perceives the sperm as "foreign" and produces antibodies to kill it or block its passage into the uterus at the cervix. Such antibodies can be detected in the woman's blood and can also be found in cervical mucus.

As with other immunological problems that affect male infertility (see #20, p. 66), there is a method to "trick" the woman's body out of this response. It's relatively simple and often the first approach that's tried. The couple is advised to use condoms during intercourse so that no sperm enters the woman's body (this includes oral sex). Since antibodies form in direct response to the presence of sperm, it's hoped that removing the sperm will remove the antibodies. Frequent blood tests will indicate when the antibodies have dropped low enough in the woman to make it possible to slip sperm past the reaction site before more antibodies can form to destroy them.

AN IMPORTANT THING YOU CAN DO

If cervical antibodies are causing your infertility, it is important to keep using condoms through the beginning of the female partner's menstrual cycle and stop their use only on the most optimum days of ovulation. You can also try intrauterine insemination, which bypasses the cervix altogether. Some doctors may recommend using low-dose steroids, but the results have been mixed, so set a deadline for any such trials beyond which you will use other methods.

PART
FOUR

PAY ATTENTION TO
YOUR LIFESTYLE

#28

USE ALCOHOL SPARINGLY

We have all heard about the effects of alcohol consumption on women who are already pregnant and the damage it can do to a fetus. But since ancient times, it has been known that alcohol causes not only birth defects but also miscarriage. If you have experienced repeated miscarriages and drink, even socially, it's best to stop altogether.

In addition, alcohol consumption in women may change their hormonal environment since alcohol affects the liver's ability to cleanse itself of hormonal debris. Subclinical amounts of different hormones and toxins can accumulate, throwing the whole axis slightly off kilter. Alcohol consumption is also known to decrease the vitamin B complex in both men and women.

In men, alcohol abuse can lower sperm production; extreme alcohol use (more than five drinks a day) can cause impotence or the failure to sustain an erection, as well as a temporary inability to ejaculate if an erection does occur, due to decreased sensation in the penis. Alcohol affects the liver in men, too, and allows small amounts of female hormones to accumulate, which, in turn, can suppress sperm production as well as decrease overall potency. Alcohol also increases the release of prolactin, which adversely affects sperm production.

Many animal studies over the years have shown that males who are given alcohol produce fewer, smaller, and weaker offspring than those sired by males who had no alcohol. Human studies within the last few years have found that the babies of fathers who drank as few as two drinks a day in the month prior to conception weighed 6.5 ounces less than other babies. These findings held fast even when the mothers neither drank nor smoked.

AN IMPORTANT THING YOU CAN DO

Couples who are trying to conceive should stop drinking altogether. This would be especially good advice for men with lowered sperm counts and erection or potency problems, for women who cannot maintain pregnancies, and for both men and women with hormonal imbalances. Many early miscarriages go undetected when they occur close to the time of an expected menstrual cycle. Even just one or two drinks a day can make a difference in some people.

#29

STOP SMOKING

Smoking—both active and passive—has an impact on the entire body, not just the lungs. Carbon monoxide and other chemicals from smoke can saturate brain cells, decrease oxygen levels in the blood, constrict blood vessels and deprive them of oxygen, reduce vitamin levels (especially antioxidants like vitamin C), cause skin aging and tissue atrophy in fine reproductive areas, and in general make the whole body sluggish and semitoxic.

Studies show that women who smoke have a 25 percent reduced fertility rate within the first year of trying to conceive when compared with nonsmoking women. When smoking is stopped, fertility returns to normal rates.

Common characteristics of babies born to mothers who smoke are low birth weights, retarded growth, premature birth, and decreased lung size. Lower IQs and learning disabilities are found more often in the school-age children of smoking parents. Passive smoke in the home increases chronic respiratory infections and susceptibility to illness in general in infants.

In men, cigarette smoking is implicated in both decreased sperm counts and lower sperm quality, probably due
to decreased oxygen in the blood and tissues. There is also
preliminary evidence of birth defects in the children of men
who smoke. The most vulnerable time for men is during
the three-month period before conception when sperm is
being produced.

AN IMPORTANT THING YOU CAN DO

When you are trying to become parents, it's important that
you both quit smoking altogether, because smoking as few as
two cigarettes a day can cause problems. Try to avoid prolonged exposure to smoke-filled environments, which is the
equivalent of smoking two cigarettes.

#30

STOP DRUG USE

Recreational drug use and pregnancy don't mix. Here's what is known about some of the more popular drugs and their impact on your fertility.

MARIJUANA

Marijuana use became popular during the 1960s and 1970s and is still a popular drug with people in their childbearing years. But when it comes to a negative impact on fertility, you should assume that marijuana carries all of the risks and side effects of cigarette smoking—and then some!

Tetrahydrocannabinol (THC) is the principal active ingredient in marijuana. It enters the bloodstream quickly, goes to the brain, and lodges in the body's fatty tissue—sometimes for months after just one use. Because women have more fat than men, THC is excreted more slowly by women. Marijuana smoking is known to cause fetal oxygen deprivation (hypoxia) in utero, which can cause brain damage.

In men, marijuana use is implicated in both lower sperm counts and chromosomally damaged sperm, so that birth defects are possible in the children of fathers who use the drug. Some substances in marijuana lodge in the testicles. Marijuana use also increases the level of prolactin in the blood, thus blocking hormonal messengers and decreasing sperm production. Frequent use decreases male sex drive.

When you are trying to conceive, it's essential that you preserve your fertility by stopping all marijuana use.

COCAINE

Cocaine became the popular "upscale" drug in the 1980s, and quickly took over (in the form of cheap crack cocaine) as the drug of choice in many inner cities. An estimated 5 million people in their childbearing years are habitual cocaine users. While little research had been done on the impact of cocaine use on fertility and childbearing up until that time, the medical community has since seen what this drug can actually do "in the field." Its effects are devastating.

As a stimulant, cocaine sharply increases blood pressure and heart rate, and can cause immediate or delayed spontaneous abortions because it constricts blood vessels. It causes a wide range of massive birth defects (depending on the stage of fetal growth when the mother ingested it), as well as brain damage and permanent learning disabilities. Since a woman doesn't even miss her period until she is fourteen days pregnant, cocaine use in women who are attempting to become pregnant is utterly self-defeating. In women who are already pregnant, sudden onset of premature labor is common with cocaine use, as well as placental separation, which threatens the baby's oxygen supply and therefore its life. Unfortunately, stillbirths are common when mothers use cocaine.

In men, cocaine can raise body temperature and damage sperm. Chronic use suppresses the appetite through its effects on the brain's central nervous system, which leads to malnutrition and hormonal imbalances that, in turn, affect sperm production.

The use of cocaine (and amphetamines) is reputed to increase libido and prolong erections, but this may be a mistaken interpretation of the elevated energy levels, restlessness, and agitation that accompany it and which cause a temporary surge of hormone release from the adrenal glands.

Cocaine use has no place in the lives of couples trying to conceive.

OTHER RECREATIONAL DRUGS

Hallucinatory drugs (LSD and PCP), amphetamines, "downers" (codeine and quaaludes), and narcotics such as the opium derivatives heroin and morphine increase prolactin levels in the blood. This interferes with hormonal production in both men and women. It throws off women's menstrual cycles and impairs men's sperm production and sex drive.

OVER-THE-COUNTER DRUGS

Many people don't realize that over-the-counter drugs often contain the same chemical compounds as prescription drugs, only in lesser quantities. You shouldn't use appetite suppressants containing phenylpropanolamine when you are trying to conceive for the same reasons that you shouldn't use amphetamines. (They constrict blood vessels that theoretically could have an adverse impact on fertility.) If you regularly take any over-the-counter drugs, even aspirin, mention this use to your infertility specialist.

AN IMPORTANT THING YOU CAN DO

If you use drugs, even occasionally, it's imperative that you stop while you are trying to become parents.

#31

FINE-TUNE YOUR NUTRITION
AND EXERCISE

Nutrition and exercise also affect fertility. Too much or too little of both appears to cause problems.

Many factors affect ovulation in women and sperm production in men, including extremes of body fat in either direction. Anorexic women and female athletes with high muscle composition often stop ovulating and menstruating. Female athletes who are infertile, even though they are taking fertility drugs, can often reverse their infertility by switching from jogging to light walking, for instance.

Male athletes who wear tight athletic supports, work out in very hot weather, or engage in prolonged athletics that raise their body temperature experience reduced sperm counts. Using hot tubs, Jacuzzis, and saunas can have the same effect, as well as damage an early embryo in a woman who is pregnant. All of these activities can raise the body's inner core temperature quite rapidly to 102 to 103 degrees Fahrenheit, where negative effects have been seen.

Obese women (those who are 20 percent over their ideal

weight for their height) also compromise their ovulation pat-terns. Fat cells produce more estrogen, and increased estrogen can alter the fine balance of a woman's hormonal axis.

Nutrition is an area where moderation is obviously re-quired. If you are underweight or overweight and are having trouble conceiving, gradually bringing yourself closer to the mid-ranges might help you become pregnant. Crash or severe liquid diets, however, will do far more harm than good. Severe caloric restrictions reduce sperm counts in men and stop ovulation in women.

There have been a handful of interesting studies on nu-trition and fertility. One study found that a mixture of vita-min C, calcium, magnesium, and manganese given to twenty men with a condition called spermagglutination (sperm clumps together and cannot swim normally), which had rendered them infertile, cured the condition within sixty days and enabled them to impregnate their wives. (A control group of seven men with the same condition and accompanying infertility were not given the vitamin C preparation and their infertility persisted.) Vitamin C not only reversed the spermagglutination in test sub-jects, but also raised their sperm counts by 53 percent. This study group was small, but the findings were significant. There appears to be some interaction between sperm physiology and the vitamin C–mineral preparation.

In a study of fourteen women with unexplained infertil-ity, high doses of vitamin B_6 had a marked positive impact. The women, ranging in age from twenty-three to thirty-one, had been infertile from eighteen months to seven years. All had premenstrual syndrome (PMS) in common. One hundred to 800 milligrams of B_6 were administered to alleviate the PMS. Twelve of the fourteen women not only became preg-nant, but their progesterone levels increased. Eleven preg-nancies occurred within the first six months, with one woman conceiving twice; one within the seventh month; and the last during the eleventh month of the study. As with the vitamin

C–minerals study, this test group was small, and the results were fascinating.

Vitamin B₆ and folate (another member of the B family) are often deficient in women who have taken birth control pills. Smoking reduces the body's store of vitamin C by as much as half. Alcohol intake reduces the entire B complex, and also creates deficiencies across the board and toxic accumulations of fat-soluble vitamins in the livers of people who both drink and take vitamins regularly.

A word of caution, however, is necessary regarding vitamin self-dosing. Mega doses of vitamins can do more harm than good. For instance, dosages of B₆ much above 150 milligrams (the ranges used in the above-mentioned study) cause some kinds of peripheral nerve damage. In addition, high doses of vitamins A and D can cause damage to adults and growing embryos. The B vitamins also work in tandem with one another and can create deficiencies in some as the levels of others are increased.

When it comes to exercise, moderation is key, too. Find the line between being an overweight couch potato and an Olympic trainee. For women who do conceive, raising the core body temperature above 102 degrees Fahrenheit can cause damage to an early embryo, as well as a miscarriage. Keep vigorous exercise routines to fifteen-minute intervals with cool-down periods in between. Learn to monitor your pulse rate during aerobic workouts. (Pulse rates should not exceed 140 beats per minute for any length of time.) Do not exercise in overly hot or humid weather. Consider adding yoga to your exercise regime. Yoga trains the body in flexibility, and its deep breathing discipline will surely come in handy if you do become pregnant and choose a natural birthing method such as Lamaze.

Women with infertility problems due to repeated miscarriages, incompetent cervix, or abnormal bleeding episodes should consult their doctors before exercising at all, as should any woman with a history of cardiac irregularities, diabetes, hypertension, anemia, or thyroid disorders. Women who experienced very fast labor or retarded fetal growth in previous pregnancies should also consult their doctors about exercise when trying to conceive.

AN IMPORTANT THING YOU CAN DO

Many states license naturopathic physicians or allow them to practice under the licenses of other alternative health-care providers like chiropractors. Naturopathic physicians, who have the same medical training as mainstream M.D.'s, use natural sources for their remedies and treatments. They are far more knowledgeable about vitamins and nutrition than most traditional doctors, who focus primarily on pathological conditions. If you are considering a course of high-dose vitamin therapy, try to do it under the care of a medical professional with some expertise in the subject. Many OB-GYNs won't know a lot about the more subtle aspects of vitamin therapy for infertility.

#32

Beware of Chemical Toxins

Chemicals are all around us, and some are more toxic than others. Of the hundreds of thousands of chemicals that we are exposed to daily in our work and home environments, relatively few have been studied for reproductive hazards.

Some chemicals seem to lodge in the testicles and ovaries and wreak reproductive havoc the same way that radiation does, either by damaging the sperm or eggs directly or by rearranging their DNA, thereby producing birth defects in the children of exposed parents. Reproductive toxins can alter hormone production in both men and women and cause temporary or permanent sterility.

The metals boron, lead, lithium, manganese, mercury, cadmium, arsenic, and antimony have been found to kill or deform sperm, cause impotence, affect libido, cause premature or delayed ejaculation or impair erections, reduce sperm volume and motility, and decrease the ability to have an orgasm.

In women, these metals are known to cause miscarriages, lodge in the ovaries and create menstrual cycle irregularities, impair the hypothalamus and pituitary, cause vascular changes, and impair embryo implantation in the uterus. Cadmium in particular is associated with implantation difficulties, which may account for the 25 percent reduced fertility in women who smoke. There are 30 micrograms of cadmium in one pack of cigarettes!

Exposures to these metals are associated with landfills, welding, jewelry making, and smelting. Others at risk of exposure include people who are regularly exposed to the following: truck, bus, or automobile exhausts; the manufacture of weather- and fire-proofing materials; ceramics, glass, or porcelain production; textile manufacturing; printing, dyeing, painting, photography, wood finishing, or leather tanning; some electrical apparatus and electroplating processes; insecticides; fungicides; and battery production.

Other chemicals that cause reproductive problems include Agent Orange (dioxin); industrial solvents and formaldehyde; polychlorinated biphenyls (PCBs) and polybrominated biphenyls (PBBs); and herbicides, insecticides, and fungicides like carbaryl, dibromochloropropane (DBCP), DDT, 2,4-D, ethylene dibromide (EDB), epichlorohydrin, and kepone (chlordecone).

Reproductive problems have also been found in health-care workers exposed to anesthetic gases: anesthesiologists, nurse-practitioners and operating-room personnel, dentists, hygienists, and veterinary workers. Difficulties observed include an increase in miscarriages and birth defects, infertility in men (without sperm damage), and hormonal problems in women through the hypothalamus-pituitary-ovarian axis. Most of these problems appear temporary and reversible if job changes are made. In addition, hairdressers are exposed to a wide variety of inhalants that are suspect.

AN IMPORTANT THING YOU CAN DO

If you are unsuccessfully trying to conceive and work in any of the professions mentioned above, investigate the chemicals you are using and try to protect yourself or temporarily change jobs. Couples who live near landfills or who have neighbors with metal-working shops next door might want to have their water tested to detect the presence of metals and industrial chemicals.

#33

LEARN ABOUT
ELECTROMAGNETIC FIELDS

Electromagnetic fields (EMFs) is the term used to describe that portion of the electromagnetic spectrum called non-ionizing radiation. Non-ionizing radiation is capable of producing a range of biological effects but is considered too low-powered to knock electrons off of their cellular orbits (which is what can cause genetic mutations), unlike ionizing radiation such as X-ray or nuclear devices. The non-ionizing bands encompass the earth's natural magnetic fields, electric power (the extremely low frequencies), our communications systems (the radio frequencies), microwave and radar equipment (the microwave/radar frequencies), and infrared devices. The dividing line between ionizing and non-ionizing radiation is visible light.

The subject of bioeffects from electromagnetic fields on the human anatomy is extremely complex, partly because of the amount of variables involved (the frequency, wavelength, power intensity, and duration of exposure; a person's size, shape, and orientation toward the source; and the tissue type being irradiated—to name but a few); and partly because of the evolving understanding of the human anatomy as a coherent electrical system that is quite unlike the "chemical mechanistic" model we have traditionally used. How electromagnetic fields affect fertility and pregnancy is more complex still because exposures to the mother might have different parameters than to an embryo or fetus. This is in addition to the inherent differences between the male and female anatomies. A particular frequency may, for instance, have detrimental effects to sperm production, while a different frequency may adversely effect a woman's hormonal axis.

Debate has raged for years over whether human reactions to EMFs are "thermally-based"—meaning they are a by-product of tissue heating much like a microwave oven heats food—or are due to "nonthermal" effects which are biological reactions below the heating threshold. Today, nonthermal effects are presumed to be true, although the actual mechanism by which they function is not yet known.

Humans can absorb radiation in all frequencies to a greater or lesser extent but we absorb it most efficiently around the FM radio band, an area of the spectrum that has seen a tremendous increase in consumer devices within the last decade alone. Different areas of the body absorb radiation differently, however. The eyes, brain and testes are more sensitive. Body tissue also responds differently to EMFs depending on its water and mineral content.

There are well over a thousand studies worldwide investigating various aspects of EMFs, many of which have found adverse reproductive effects in both humans and animals. Studies include controlled laboratory work with animals, occupational observations, and epidemiological surveys of population groups. Reduced fertility rates, increased incidence of brain, blood, and lymphatic cancers, and birth defects have been reported in some people who live near high tension lines or who work in the electrical professions. The same bioeffects have been observed near radar installations, or among law enforcement personnel who use hand-held radar guns, as well as in a few communities living near radio and TV transmission facilities, in HAM radio operators, and CB radio users. Some studies go back to the 1940s in which reduced sperm counts were found in radar operators aboard Navy ships. Another study found an increase in Down's syndrome in children fathered by such military radar men. Two recent studies have found increases in miscarriages in magnetic resonance imaging (MRI) operators. Other studies have found increased miscarriages in diathermy operators.

Numerous animal studies have found reduced fertility, fewer uterine implantation sites, smaller liter sizes, testicular atrophy, miscarriages, lower birth weights, and birth defects in the offspring of animals exposed to different frequencies and power intensities for varying durations. Changes have been repeatedly observed in test animals' immune systems, as well as alterations to important hormones and neurotransmitters in the brain, and in calcium-ion flow at the cell's surface. Melatonin and endocrine-gland suppression have also been observed in several studies, as well as testosterone reduction in male test animals. Most studies were conducted at high-power exposures for short durations. But some were low-power studies over several generations of test animals, and detrimental effects were observed then, too. Two recent studies have found DNA damage in test animals exposed to microwave frequencies similar to those used in cellular phones.

A series of studies conducted in the 1980s and 1990s found as much as a 50 percent increase in miscarriages in women who slept under electric blankets, in electrically heated water beds or in rooms with electric ceiling cable heat. The winter months saw a steep rise in the miscarriage rates (when heat settings would be higher) than during the summer months.

Research has found more detrimental "windows" for some frequencies than for others. Windows appear to exist for the human anatomy around the electric-power frequencies and the microwave frequencies. Research has also found increases in certain chemicals that are produced during times of stress in test animals exposed to EMFs that didn't appear to be feeling especially "stressed out." Stress can exist at the subliminal level but the chemical changes can be detrimental nevertheless. Stress is known to affect fertility through the hormone balance in both men and women.

Several studies found that some frequencies at very low levels initially activated the immune system but when exposures continued, the immune system became suppressed. Some episodes of unexplained infertility, or some of the baffling antibody responses in both men and women, may eventually be traced to EMFs. Promising research on reduced melatonin production in the pituitary gland (after certain EMF exposures) may also serve to explain some infertility cases today. In the past, anything that adversely effected this area of the brain was found to have important ramifications to fertility through the ovarian axis in women, and sperm production in men.

AN IMPORTANT THING YOU CAN DO

The best EMF advice when you are trying to conceive is "prudent avoidance," meaning reduce all exposures to a minimum. Do not use electric blankets except to warm the bed before you get in. Then unplug it since current still exists in the wires whether it's on or off. Keep use of electric hair dryers, razors, and cordless/cellular phones to a minimum. Keep arm's length from any computer screen. Rearrange work space so that you are not exposed to cross-fields from printers, copy machines, faxes, etc. Be aware of co-workers' equipment too. The highest exposures often come from the back and sides of machines.

While watching TV at home, stay at least 8 feet from the set. Try to position electric appliances—stoves, ovens, microwaves, refrigerators, washers/dryers, etc.—a slight distance from the work area where you stand. EMF's fall off rapidly with distance. Just 1 to 3 feet can make a significant difference.

PART FIVE

STACK THE FERTILITY DECK IN YOUR FAVOR

#34

LEARN HOW TO PREDICT OVULATION

Knowing when your fertility is at its monthly peak will greatly increase your ability to become pregnant. It is not unusual for a fertility counselor to discover that timing alone makes the difference for some couples.

BASAL BODY TEMPERATURE

Timing is an essential aspect of becoming pregnant. During each monthly cycle—even with unimpaired fertility—there is roughly a 25 percent chance of becoming pregnant. So being able to gauge your optimum days is important. One way to tell is to keep a record of the woman's basal body temperature (BBT). Charting your temperature is one of the first things that an infertility specialist will ask you to do. This simple test, done at home, will aid in the evaluation process.

Sperm can fertilize an egg for an estimated twenty-four to forty-eight hours after ejaculation. The egg is capable of being fertilized for an average of twelve to twenty-four hours after ovulation. There are variations, however: In a few cases, sexual relations up to seven days prior to a rise in BBT (and therefore ovulation) have resulted in pregnancy.

Recording your BBT requires more consistency than skill. All you need is a regular thermometer (used orally or rectally) or new BBT thermometers are available. If you prefer, you can use a more expensive digital model that records subtle temperature changes. Charts can be obtained from your doctor or you can make your own. It's best to keep the thermometer and chart by your bedside and to record your temperature first thing in the morning *before* getting out of bed.

To make a temperature chart, use regular or graph paper. Note the month at the top of the paper and list days 1 through 28 (or however long your regular cycle is) across the bottom. This chart reflects your period cycle, *not* the specific month. Starting at the top on the left side, record temperatures beginning at 99.0 down to 97.0. On the first day of your period, start recording your morning temperature. Here's what an average monthly chart might look like:

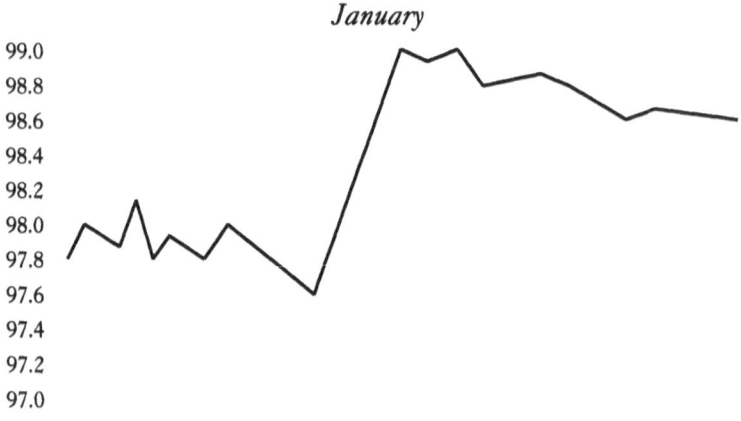

January

Day: 1 2 3 4 5 6 7 8 9 10 11 12 13 14 15 16 17 18 19 20 21 22 23 24 25 26 27 28

Just before ovulation occurs, your temperature may drop surprisingly lower than the normal 98.6 degrees Fahrenheit to a range between 97.2 and 97.4 degrees. (The drop is caused by the increase of estrogen needed to release the egg during ovulation within the next few days.) If your menstrual cycle is twenty-eight days, you should notice your temperature rise around days 12 to 14 to over 98 degrees (as levels of progesterone increase). Ovulation will already have occurred then. Some women will experience a rise in body temperature to 98.8, 99.0, or higher, and their temperatures will remain elevated until menstruation begins. Other women will see their temperatures drop a few days before their period begins, which might indicate a too-short corpus luteum phase. On the chart each month, also note the days on which you had intercourse or perhaps experienced a rise in temperature due to illness such as colds or flu. Not everyone benefits from keeping a BBT chart. Some women maintain a constant body temperature throughout their cycles even though they are ovulating regularly.

The time to become pregnant is during ovulation. Fertility specialists recommend sexual intercourse every thirty-six to forty-eight hours during the time when your BBT begins to drop, about three to four days before ovulation, as well as for two to three days after your BBT begins to rise. (It's important to understand that these are just guidelines and are not meant to lock you into an "intercourse-on-schedule" routine, which many couples say kills spontaneity in lovemaking.)

CERVICAL MUCUS AND VAGINAL CHANGES

Another way to help predict when ovulation is about to occur is to note changes in your cervical mucus about the time when temperature drops and estrogen levels surge. Cervical mucus is normally cloudy and thick, but just prior to ovulation its texture becomes thinner, its color is clearer, and there is more of it. These changes are the result of the body's alteration in pH to create a more hospitable environment for sperm. There are other physical changes you can learn to recognize as ovulation approaches, including a feeling in the vaginal area of additional lubrication, swelling, and fullness.

Ovulation Predictor Test Kits

A relatively recent innovation for couples trying to conceive is the ovulation predictor test kit, several brands of which are available without a prescription. The kits measure the presence of the hormone LH, which rises just before ovulation occurs. A dipstick turns blue when placed in urine. Such kits can predict ovulation accurately within twenty to forty-four hours. While more accurate than keeping a BBT chart or trying to gauge cervical mucus changes, their drawback is the added expense—as much as thirty dollars a month.

AN IMPORTANT THING YOU CAN DO

Learn to identify your most fertile days by keeping a temperature chart, identifying changes in cervical mucus, or using ovulation predictor test kits. Sometimes it's best not to rely on only one method but to combine all three: keep a BBT chart, notice changes in cervical mucus, and supplement with an ovulation predictor kit. Combined efforts will improve accuracy.

#35

SPACE YOUR EJACULATIONS

Men with low sperm counts are well advised to refrain from sexual activity during the first half of their mate's menstrual cycle, in order to build up enough sperm to maximize the chances of conceiving. But abstaining for seven days or longer may do more harm than good, because the gain in sperm count will be offset by the increase in aged sperm cells, which have lower potential for fertilization.

During the woman's most fertile days, it is best to have sexual intercourse every thirty-six to forty-eight hours. More frequent intercourse can depress the sperm count into the too-low range; with less frequent intercourse, you run the risk of missing the fertile period completely.

AN IMPORTANT THING YOU CAN DO

Discuss timing and how to space sexual activity to your best advantage with your fertility specialist. Men who chronically ejaculate prematurely can collect their semen for near-future use in artificial insemination.

PART SIX

INVESTIGATE TODAY'S HIGH-TECH INFERTILITY SOLUTIONS

#36

LOOK INTO SOME REPRODUCTIVE OPTIONS

Sometimes conceiving a child can only be accomplished with a little more help from the medical community. Artificial insemination is the least complicated, most tried-and-true method of achieving successful pregnancies thwarted by low sperm count and cervical mucus disorders. It is the oldest method employed to solve infertility problems; early attempts in humans can be traced as far back as the 1790s.

There are two basic categories: artificial insemination by the husband (AIH) and artificial insemination by a donor (AID). In both methods, a small plastic tube is used to place the sperm close to the cervical canal or uterus, thus bypassing the vagina. Depending on the cause of infertility, overall pregnancy success rates for artificial insemination can be similar to those of fertile couples.

A small plastic cup is often positioned over the cervix after insemination; sometimes the sperm can be injected through an opening in it. The sperm are thus held and protected for several hours as they try to penetrate the cervical mucus and enter the uterus.

When cervical antibodies are found to be the cause of infertility (see page 90), artificial insemination is done directly into the uterus. But because there is an increased risk of infection and painful uterine contractions, this procedure is less often recommended and is not performed routinely.

Couples who choose artificial insemination will be asked to record their BBTs or to use ovulation predictor kits to test their urine for LH. Insemination will be done midcycle, just prior to ovulation. Ultrasound and blood tests can also be used to determine ovulation, but these procedures are more expensive. Women who do not ovulate or who ovulate irregularly may take fertility-enhancing medication during the insemination time span.

AN IMPORTANT THING YOU CAN DO

Ask your doctor for the names of couples who have used artificial insemination. Make a list of questions to ask in advance, and follow through with phone calls.

#37

EXPLORE ARTIFICIAL INSEMINATION USING THE HUSBAND'S SPERM (AIH)

Men who have low sperm counts, severe premature ejaculatory disorders, retrograde ejaculation, hypospadias, sperm that either clumps together or is too abundant, or semen that is either too thick or too thin are all good candidates for having children of their own with the aid of artificial insemination (AIH). Through the use of laboratory techniques that can separate and wash sperm samples, AIH makes the most out of the sperm that's available, asking it to do the least amount of work.

Most infertility specialists will ask their clients to come to the office to give sperm samples. The man is asked to masturbate into a sterile glass jar. Sperm is then quickly scanned under a microscope for quality and character, and implantation is done within a half hour. Men who collect their sperm samples at home are asked to masturbate into a sterile glass jar, to keep it warm by holding it close to the body, and to deliver it to the infertility specialist's office within an hour.

For the woman, the procedure resembles a regular gynecological examination and Pap test. A speculum is inserted through the vagina and a syringe is used to inject the sperm into the cervical canal. A small silicone cap may be placed over the cervix, and the woman is asked to lie quietly for fifteen to thirty minutes. After six hours, she can remove the cervical cap herself at home.

Success rates vary, but in select cases approximately 30 percent will conceive within the first month, 50 to 70 percent by the third month, and 80 percent by the sixth month.

There is also a physician-directed, at-home method for AIH that offers some advantages over in-office procedures, including less cost, fresh semen samples, and considerably less psychological stress, which can adversely affect ovulation. It also returns a sense of personal power to couples already in a frustrating situation beyond their choice and control.

The procedure is almost identical to the office technique. The woman positions a silicone cup over her cervix while her mate masturbates into a sterile glass jar. They then allow fifteen to twenty minutes for the semen to liquefy. The man then draws it up into a plastic syringe and inserts it through an opening in the silicone cup, slowly depressing the pump. The cup is left in place for six hours.

It is recommended that a couple repeat this technique two to three times per menstrual cycle, at midcycle. Keeping a BBT chart and knowing how to judge cervical mucus changes will help best to determine when a woman is most fertile.

One study found a reduced overall success rate (around 53 percent) for the at-home method, so couples who are anxious to become pregnant, or who are facing biological time-clock pressures or health issues, may not want to try this approach for an indefinite period.

AN IMPORTANT THING YOU CAN DO

Determine which approach works best for you. Keep in mind that "best" doesn't necessarily mean the most convenient. Set a deadline for at-home procedures beyond which, if pregnancy hasn't occurred, you will try more "inconvenient" office procedures.

#38

FIND OUT ABOUT
DONOR SPERM (AID)

A couple may choose to use artificial insemination with donor sperm (AID) when the male partner's sperm cannot be used because there isn't enough, or there are genetic complications to consider; there has been exposure to toxins such as dioxin; the partners are infertile together, or have Rh (blood) incompatibilities; or prolonged infertility exists without explanation.

Ten to twenty thousand children conceived through AID are born each year in the United States, and those numbers are rising.

There are several advantages to using AID. First, there is at least one biological parent: the mother. Second, the physical characteristics of the father (eye and hair color, height, weight, racial background) can be matched to the donor's. In fact, some sperm banks offer a wide variety of international donors, which improves the odds of matching the father's physical characteristics. Third, it is possible to segregate donor sperm into several batches for future use, thereby allowing parents to have more children who are truly biologically related siblings. Fourth, prescreening techniques for AID can eliminate the possibility of genetic disorders like Tay-Sachs (which primarily affects people of Jewish descent).

AID is also a way around the general backlog and delays of adoption agencies. A biological mother will not show up later in the child's life, nor will a surrogate challenge parental rights. And since sperm donors are not told what happens to their samples, there's little chance that a biological father will turn up, although the legalities of reproductive law continue to evolve in unpredictable ways. AID is a reasonably safe alternative for women who choose to have children outside of traditional family models.

There are disadvantages to AID as well. The main drawback, of course, is that the couple won't know who the donor is. Many times his genetic background is not thoroughly screened, especially in small communities where donations are made to private doctors' offices. Most reputable sperm banks try to be thorough, but there are no guarantees. A couple must sign a consent form accepting responsibility for the child despite its physical condition. Although the incidence of genetically transmitted disorders is not greater among children conceived through AID than among the "regular" population, an increase is theoretically possible as AID is used more frequently.

Another significant disadvantage is the slight chance of acquiring a sexually transmitted disease, including HIV, from the donor semen. Make sure that all donors are thoroughly screened for sexually transmitted diseases to minimize this risk.

You can find ways around these problems, however.

Genetic screening can be expensive, but any couple considering AID should make sure that the sperm bank or administering physician has conducted a thorough genetic background check of the donor. This will include a careful family history for any genetic difficulties, and if any seem likely, a genetic karyotype (photograph of chromosome arrangement within a cell) should be done.

It is not out of line to request a copy of the donor's family medical history since this will certainly be the baseline for health-care considerations throughout your child's lifetime. Request that the donor fill out a family history worksheet compiled by the physician, or you can get a form through your local March of Dimes chapter.

Ask a lot of questions about the sperm bank's sources and procedures. Who are its typical donors? Are donors typically from a large or small community? (Large communities are less likely to have related parents but more likely to have sexually transmitted diseases.) What are the ages of donors? What kind of genetic screening does the sperm bank do? What kinds of physical screening are done for infections? Is the sperm fresh or frozen? (Frozen sperm is often better screened.)

Your doctor will more than likely be using the services of a sperm bank. This offers some advantages over private, fresh sperm donations from small communities, including the fact that sperm banks screen and test donors more thoroughly.

Before sperm banks freeze samples, they are checked for venereal infections, HIV, damage, and overall quality. In addition, donors are checked for disease and many genetic disorders. There is some concern about the length of time that sperm can remain frozen. Genetic damage could occur in time, although children born from frozen samples have proved as healthy as naturally conceived children. At the present, the main drawback of using frozen sperm appears to be a lessened success rate for impregnation than with fresh samples. Fresh sperm can live up to forty-eight hours after insemination while frozen sperm, which may have reduced motility, live only about twenty-four hours. It is therefore more important to accurately time insemination to ovulation. Studies show that when this is done, the success rate rises to that of fresh sperm inseminations.

AN IMPORTANT THING YOU CAN DO

Find out which sperm bank your doctor uses. Call and ask questions about its health-screening techniques.

#39

FIND OUT IF YOU'RE A CANDIDATE FOR
IN VITRO FERTILIZATION (IVF)

In vitro fertilization (IVF) is the most complicated, costly, and controversial of all the attempts to address infertility, raising notions of science gone amok in the laboratory, creating a class of test-tube babies for some mechanistic, futuristic non-humanitarian use. The procedure, however, holds genuine promise and hope for couples who cannot have children any other way.

The concept is deceptively simple: Remove an egg from the mother, mix it with sperm until it is fertilized, then put the fertilized egg back into the uterus where it will become a healthy baby as if there had been no interference whatsoever. The reality, however, is quite different. Nature's work, it turns out, is far more delicate and ingenious than the hands of man, no matter how skilled. Maintaining the proper hormone balance, removing the egg at its exact moment of maturity, and nurturing the fertilization process must all be achieved in this procedure—a tall order.

Women with badly scarred fallopian tubes or endometriosis are the most likely candidates for this technique. But the procedure is very expensive and may take a prolonged period of time, and the success rate is low. Any couple venturing into these waters needs strong commitment to the process. In addition, the techniques vary from clinic to clinic, and the whole procedure is still in the experimental stages.

To be considered for this approach, the woman will need at least one functioning ovary and her mate must produce viable sperm. Corrective microsurgery may be necessary if the woman's ovaries are scarred or injured, or if the man has any duct or transport problems. Hormone therapy and fertility drugs may also be required.

A full fertility workup is mandatory and any possibility of infections must be eliminated. The ovaries must be surgically accessible; sperm will be thoroughly analyzed. Sometimes a laparoscopy is done to evaluate the ovaries. Once all these tests are complete, IVF can be tried.

The first phase involves careful attention to the production and maturing of the eggs. Fertility drugs are administered to mature more than one egg in a cycle in the hope that if more than one is fertilized and implanted the chances of a successful pregnancy are increased.

The woman will be asked to go to the clinic daily for blood tests to measure hormonal changes and for ultrasound scanning of the maturing eggs. When ovulation is imminent, a team of surgeons will be waiting on twenty-four-hour standby since ovulation can happen at any time. Once an egg is released from the ovary it cannot be retrieved, so the whole process is bumped into the next menstrual cycle.

The mature eggs are removed through laparoscopy, and the retrieval success rate is near 90 percent. Each egg is placed in a culture dish, examined by a tissue specialist, and treated with a special medium that varies from clinic to clinic. The woman often remains in the hospital recovering from the laparoscopy and waiting for the implantation, which often takes place within forty hours.

The second phase, fertilization, is about to begin. While the woman undergoes the removal of her eggs, her mate collects sperm through masturbation. His sperm is separated from the semen by using centrifugal force. It is then capacitated, treated, washed, and resuspended in a fresh liquid medium.

Each egg is then combined with approximately 100,000 to 200,000 sperm and placed in an incubator for twelve hours. They are then examined under a microscope to see if fertilization has taken place. If it has, the cell is allowed to divide several times—a general indication of good health—and is considered ready for implantation after four to eight cell divisions.

The third phase is about to begin, and it is the most hazardous one for the fertilized zygote. Successful implantation is the most difficult and complex aspect of IVF. The skill of the IVF team counts a great deal, and, even in experienced hands, the success rates hover around only 20 percent for each attempt.

Before implantation, progesterone shots are administered to the woman to help prepare the uterus hormonally. The fertilized eggs are drawn up into a long, thin tube containing some of the culture medium and then inserted into her uterus vaginally through the cervical opening. Her partner is often present. The woman is advised to rest for several hours at the hospital and for two days at home. During the following week she may undergo daily blood tests to check progesterone levels.

Because of the complex hormonal interaction between the uterus and ova within the first twelve weeks, one-third of all embryos will spontaneously abort; an additional 10 to 15 percent will be lost later. In the final analysis only about 10 percent of women who undergo IVF will have successful embryos implanted and deliver a live baby. Although this success rate is low when weighed against the incredible expenditure of time, energy, expectations, and cost, the couples who become parents usually consider it worth the effort. Another way to think about it is this. The chances of becoming successfully pregnant for normally fertile couples in any given menstrual cycle is itself only about 25 percent.

As this procedure is perfected, the success rate will improve, and the costs, which now average around five thousand dollars per cycle, will decrease.

AN IMPORTANT THING YOU CAN DO

Every in vitro clinic has its own protocol. Success rates can vary widely between clinics. Reputable clinics are registered with The American Society for Reproductive Medicine, which sets standards and ethical guidelines as a prerequisite for membership. Contact them before signing up with a clinic (see #1, page 7, for address). The clinic "closest to home" may not always be the best choice. The same criteria for choosing an infertility specialist apply to in vitro clinics too. Clearly in vitro fertilization is complex, costly, time and energy consuming and involves major medical procedures for the female partner. It is important that you have clear determination before you set out on this course. Ask your surgeon what his or her success rates are. Decide in advance how many cycles of in vitro you are willing to try.

#40

KEEP UP WITH THE LATEST IN VITRO APPROACHES

Two new approaches have been added to IVF attempts, and both are exciting to specialists in the field. One involves freezing the embryos after fertilization for later use. This reduces the amount of surgical procedures needed since many eggs can be removed at one time. The repeated hormonal therapy is also reduced. The other involves using ultrasound to locate the mature eggs, which are then removed with a long, thin suction needle inserted through the abdomen under local anesthesia, instead of laparoscopy, which is more invasive and requires general anesthesia. Fertilization can then proceed in the test tube, or the eggs and sperm can be washed, treated, and simultaneously returned to the uterus (through the cervix), where fertilization takes place. This latter method eliminates most of the complicated laboratory work and the whole approach can greatly simplify IVF. Success rates are comparable to those of the "older" techniques.

AN IMPORTANT THING YOU CAN DO

Keep up with the latest in vitro research by talking to your doctor and consulting medical journals.

#41

EXPLORE GAMETE INTRAFALLOPIAN TRANSFER (GIFT)

In gamete intrafallopian transfer (GIFT), the mature egg is removed from the ovary; after both the egg and sperm are washed and treated, they are introduced through a laparoscope directly into the fallopian tube, where fertilization occurs naturally. One advantage of this approach is lower failure rates than those associated with implantation directly into the uterus. If a fertilized egg can travel the natural course of the fallopian tube, doctors believe the uterus will be in more precise hormonal harmony when implantation occurs.

GIFT is a promising solution for men with low sperm counts or delivery disorders since the sperm bypasses the vagina, cervix, and uterus. Success rates are low, however, and the procedure is done at only a few major medical centers. Nevertheless, GIFT is a promising alternative to IVF.

AN IMPORTANT THING YOU CAN DO

Find out if a specialist in your area is doing GIFT procedures. Make an appointment to speak with that person.

#42

BECOME INFORMED ABOUT SURROGACY

A surrogate mother is artificially inseminated with the sperm of a man who is not her spouse. She carries the baby to term and surrenders it to the man and his mate after birth. The advantages to the couple include the biological linkage of at least one parent to the child. Often the surrogate mother shares her pregnancy process with the couple, which is important for family bonding. The couple pays all of her expenses plus a fee ranging from five thousand to thirty thousand dollars.

Although biblical references to surrogate mothers go as far back as two thousand years, surrogacy is today one of the most controversial answers to infertility. It's not likely that the legal uncertainties involved will be easily solved with one or two court rulings. To guarantee legal custody, the couple adopts the child after its birth, because in many states the paternity of the biological father is not secure. Under the law, he can be considered a sperm donor rather than a legal custodian.

To avoid potential problems, it is best to use a surrogacy clinic supervised by doctors and lawyers rather than well-intentioned laypeople. Genetic counseling and family history is just as important for surrogate mothers as for sperm donors.

AN IMPORTANT THING YOU CAN DO

Search for a team of people who can provide medical, legal, and psychological support. Investigate several centers. Ask about their criteria for selecting appropriate surrogates. What medical and psychological screening is done? Keep in mind that a responsible surrogate will want to know, and is entitled to know, as much as she can about you, too.

#43

EDUCATE YOURSELF ABOUT EMBRYO TRANSFER

Embryo transfer is a form of surrogate mothering. A woman agrees to the fertilization of her eggs with the sperm of a man who is not her spouse. The embryo is then transferred to the uterus of the man's mate. If all goes well, the couple can in essence experience the birth of their own child who is genetically related to the father.

This procedure is still experimental and, like in vitro fertilization, it's complicated. Success rates are low, but there have been successful pregnancies. Tremendous controversy surrounds post-menopausal women who use embryo transfer techniques today. Some countries are even considering legislation against it.

Embryo transfer is a viable option for women whose ovaries don't produce eggs, but who want children and to experience the birthing process, and who are not comfortable with the idea of using a surrogate. Other candidates include women with damaged fallopian tubes or those who may pass on genetic disorders.

AN IMPORTANT THING YOU CAN DO

Find a doctor who has performed this procedure. Ask detailed questions about what kinds of hormonal changes to expect and what kinds of medications will be recommended. If you are post-menopausal and considering this procedure, know that it will kick your entire body back into high hormonal activity.

#44

INVESTIGATE ADOPTION

Many couples who consider adoption would like to see themselves reflected in the children they choose: it's an emotional fact of parenting. White couples primarily want white babies; black couples want black babies; while those couples who have made mixed-race adoptions have recently come under criticism from various racial groups, to the surprise of many. Foreign adoptions have so far been less problematic on such issues of principle but the area is rife with difficulties.

However, because of the large number of infertile couples and the small number of illegitimate births due to the availability of contraceptives and elective abortion, there are currently ten requests for every baby available at regular adoption agencies, where couples wait an average of five to seven years for a child after an initial application is made. (The waiting period for minority and older children is shorter.) As a result, many couples seek private adoption arrangements with individual mothers. Although these arrangements can be problematic, about half of all adoptions fall into this category, and there are attorneys who specialize in this field. Anyone considering a private adoption arrangement is well advised to seek one out. Many people choose foreign adoption services that often work in concert with U.S. embassy doctors in their country of origin to help select children.

Adoption can be expensive. Private arrangements can range between three thousand and six thousand dollars, depending on whether a couple assumes the medical costs of the mother in advance. Foreign adoption costs between five hundred and three thousand dollars for Latin American babies and about one thousand dollars for Asian children.

Because of the cost and the impediments inherent in the process, many couples opt for some of the high-tech medical solutions as a first choice today, considering adoption as a last resort. Not long ago, it used to be the other way around.

AN IMPORTANT THING YOU CAN DO

If you are positive that you want to be parents (whether there's a biological connection or not), but you want to pursue biological solutions, too, consider filing applications with adoption agencies while you are trying to become pregnant. This two-pronged approach may save you time later.

PART SEVEN

SET UP YOUR SUPPORT TEAM

#45

SEEK PSYCHOLOGICAL ALLIES

The decision to have a child is a deeply personal one between two people. Up until that time, notions of having a family are rather abstract, with both mates projecting themselves into roles of parenting and partnering. But once the decision is made, a couple can become profoundly committed to each other's health, well-being, career, genetic background, and visions of the future.

If a couple committed to becoming parents discovers they are infertile, it can be a shattering, disillusioning, heartbreaking experience, creating, in many instances, what seems to be irreconcilable distance.

Blame, mistrust, and accusations enter the picture. Sex becomes "work" rather than pleasure. Both partners can feel incompetent. There is a pervasive sense of failure and often tremendous anger and depression. In time, the pursuit of pregnancy can absorb all of your thoughts and many of your actions. It is an extraordinarily stressful time in any relationship. A woman may see her mate as uncooperative and unsupportive, while a man may resent "obligatory" sex-on-schedule. Both partners can develop new and unflattering perspectives on the other.

Infertility specialists encounter all of these emotions in those they see. The best specialists will be sensitive to your emotional and physical complexities. They will neither ignore nor over-dwell on relevant emotions. Look for someone who encourages the human side along with the hi-tech medical solutions.

Many infertility practices with busy doctors have nurse practitioners who help to answer emotional as well as medical questions. But it is also a good idea to seek short-term couple's counseling with a therapist during this period.

Many infertile couples report a significant reduction in stress, depression, and anxiety after only a few sessions with a therapist, but it's important to commit to the possibility of a longer relationship (eight to twenty sessions) since you don't know at the outset what will be enough.

Infertility can create artificial obstacles in communication between mates, often because each one is afraid of hurting the other's feelings or is too ambivalent about his or her own emotions to articulate them very well. The therapist's role is to tease apart what's important during this time from what isn't.

Be sure that the therapist has experience with infertility issues, which are unique problems that require particular short-term expertise. Though profound insights may occur during this period, you are not necessarily looking for in-depth analysis. You want a kind, effective, trained, knowledgeable troubleshooter. The therapist should have at least a master's degree in psychology, social work, counseling, or psychiatric nursing, with a special concentration in couple's infertility work. You may want to continue in-depth therapy with this person later on, but it should not be your immediate concern.

It is *not* the role of an infertility counselor to ferret out a deep-seated neurosis in your relationship or personal lives on which to blame the infertility. Any qualified counselor will presume that the infertility is medically based. The counselor's role is to help both of you to resolve marital tension during this time, to minimize relational stress, and to teach you stress-management techniques. It is imperative that you are both comfortable with this person; that you both feel validated and safe.

It is also the role of the counselor to help you decide whom to tell and when. Some people feel shame when they are unable to conceive. Friends and family members sometimes try so hard to help that they intrude on the couple's privacy. Many times infertile couples actually don't know what would be helpful from others. They can become defensive and withdrawn when too much attention is focused on their "problem," which in reality is a very private matter.

Reducing stress is another good reason for counseling. The subject of stress and infertility is controversial. Although it isn't often spoken of in medical offices, reducing stress can help the medical outcome. Well-meaning friends and family can unwittingly make the situation worse by saying things like "if you just didn't work so hard, you'd get pregnant" or "if you just relaxed more." It's easy for infertile couples to internalize these comments and blame themselves.

Stress itself is complex. What stresses one person may relax another. There is important preliminary research on various forms of externally caused physical stress responses that have little to do with mental attitude or lifestyle. Some forms of low-level electromagnetic fields, for instance, seem to create a stress response in the body, with accompanying hormonal changes. People feel perfectly relaxed, but tests show high levels of specific stress-related hormones such as adrenaline in their blood. Stress causes a cascade of chemical alterations in the body, some of which may be related to fertility.

It's important to keep the psychological aspects of infertility in perspective and to remember that there is such a thing as gross pathology, too. No amount of stress reduction is going to unblock damaged fallopian tubes. Infertility counselors invariably say that stress alone does not determine who does or does not become pregnant. Some very high-strung clients become pregnant easily; others who are very relaxed do not. If you feel that stress may be an important piece to your fertility puzzle, by all means pursue stress management with a therapist. Meditation can also help.

Resolve, Inc., in Somerville, Massachusetts, is a well-known, reputable, professional self-help organization with more than fifty chapters nationwide. They have a telephone help line to answer medical questions and can refer you to infertility specialists and counselors in your area. They also publish numerous fact sheets on various infertility tests and treatments, as well as a newsletter.

AN IMPORTANT THING YOU CAN DO

Contact Resolve, Inc., for a list of psychotherapists who specialize in infertility counseling in your area (see #1, page 8, for address and phone number). Set up interview appointments.

#46

TRY NOT TO THINK OF SEX AS "WORK"

The "work" of sex is a problem particular to infertile couples. When two people are so focused on producing a baby, their enjoyment of each other can take a backseat to when ovulation is occurring. Being tired or feeling moody must take second place to "baby time." Many couples come to resent sex-on-schedule, and consequently each other. Some have found ways around it, such as having sex anywhere but in the bedroom, making sex a playful event rather than a duty.

The mass-marketing of sex implies that everyone is born knowing how to be a good lover, which is often not the case. Many men have never even been introduced to the idea that sexually "pleasing" a woman is a worthwhile activity, and those who have been sometimes think of it in formulaic terms. Women often think that a kind of passive willingness is all that's necessary on their part. But the range of sexual expression is much larger than this and some infertile couples use what is an otherwise stressful period in their lives to explore a wider experience, gaining an intimacy they didn't have before, whether they eventually conceive or not.

Modern life is busy, and many couples feel they do not have the time (or often the inclination) to reset their priorities to include careful attention to each other's sexual needs. Often people who feel overworked would rather be on the receiving end of personal attention than on the giving end. Saying this in an honest way to your mate can be difficult, but it's certainly worth the effort, as long as the other person is on the receiving end at times, too.

When couples come up against infertility, especially when there are "ability" difficulties in men, such as impotence or premature ejaculation, time, pressure, or willingness problems feed into a whole mental picture in which things look unworkable and insolvable. Anger and confusion can become so intense that the only way to stay together is to slip into terse silence about things. Sex can get shelved in the name of loftier issues like companionship or careers. This is a common situation facing two-career couples who decide to finally have a child. Sometimes the sexual distance that works its way into busy lives can seem too great to traverse.

Below are some useful exercises designed to help not only those with sexual dysfunctions but also those feeling pressured by sex-on-demand when they want to create a child. The exercises are not meant to enhance fertility but rather to help you rediscover each other as a loving couple, as opposed to a couple obsessed with infertility solutions.

Many infertile couples report that it can take years to renew a sense of sexuality apart from baby-making efforts after the infertility battles are in the past. Depending on where you are in the infertility process, the exercises may help if incorporated into a "vacation from trying." But some couples may just feel too weary and view notions like these as anathema. The process is an individual one, and it's important not to feel pressured.

TRY THESE EXERCISES

Thanks to Masters and Johnson, the 1960s pioneer sex researchers, a whole field has developed to help call "time out" on goal-oriented, hurried sex, including its relationship to sexual dysfunction. They developed sensate focusing exercises, which in effect introduce you to your own body and what pleases you. But these exercises may not be for everyone. Do what's best for you.

There is no set duration limit for these exercises, but it is recommended that you stay with each step until you are both comfortable with it before going on to the next one. Each phase can take days, weeks, or months. The only goal here is to enjoy each other's giving and taking. These exercises are also beneficial for anyone who has not been sexually active for a while and for those whose sex lives have bogged down into unimaginative routine and boredom.

SENSATE EXERCISE I: Each partner should take turns being completely receptive to attention from the other, for fifteen to twenty minutes at a time. The other partner should explore, caress, stimulate, stroke, and massage any and every part of the body *EXCEPT* the genitals and breasts. The parts we automatically associate with sexual activity are the only off-limit areas.

The intention is to become comfortable with both giving and receiving sensual attention, and to include the whole body in sexuality rather than just specific genital sites. Vary the quality and kind of touching; use light fingertips, stroking, kneading, and rubbing. Don't use just the hands—try lips and hair, for instance.

It is also very important to understand (and be comfortable with) the fact that all sex does not have to lead to intercourse. This narrow misconception of sex = intercourse = orgasm = ejaculation, without which there is failure, is often what leads to sexual dysfunction. It helps if partners take turns initiating the activity so that neither one gets hooked on mentally keeping score of giving more than getting, which is not helpful here.

SENSATE EXERCISE 2: When you are both relaxed and comfortable with just being physically expressive with each other go on to Exercise 2. All of the activities from Exercise 1 are included here, but now the genital areas can be touched. Orgasm and penetration are off-limits, even though oral stimulation of the genitals is allowed. Stop any genital stimulation when it seems as if orgasm may occur. If it does, do not scold, feel guilty, or recriminate. Let yourselves off the hook and go back to pleasing each other.

Feedback from each partner is important in both receiving and giving. Expressing what pleases you most will transmit the kind of information that each of you needs to know about the other but may have been too timid or embarrassed to ask before now. It's the perfect opportunity to learn about yourself and let your partner know, too.

It is not necessary that everything please you. Gentle honesty counts. Keep in mind that if you tell your partner that something feels good when it doesn't because you're afraid of hurt feelings, it's more than likely that your partner will continue to repeat the activity.

SENSATE EXERCISE 3: All aspects of Exercises 1 and 2 are continued, but penetration and orgasm are included if you are both comfortable with it. Whenever anyone feels unready or simply wants to stay with the other exercises, it's helpful to go back.

Benefits of the Sensate Exercises

Psychologically based impotence will probably benefit most from extended attention to Exercise 1. Creating a safe, accepting, and open environment for sensuality (not just sexuality) is up to both partners, but neither one is completely "responsible" for the other's sexual happiness.

Because impotence is so frightening and threatening, it's easy to transfer some of these feelings onto others, blaming them for what occurs in us. It's also easy to accept that blame, getting locked into solving the problem for the other person. It is always ultimately our own responsibility to learn about ourselves and to transmit this knowledge clearly to our mates.

Gaining control of premature ejaculation is helped by learning to distinguish various phases of sexual arousal. Not making intercourse the focus of sexual activity often removes the anxiety that underlies this difficulty. Using the sensate focusing exercises consistently reduces anxiety by removing the pressure to perform in any genital way. During the first exercise, many men are pleasantly surprised to find that they are able to maintain an erection for fifteen to twenty minutes without ejaculating.

When genital contact is introduced in Exercise 2, concentrating on the immediate preejaculatory period (when ejaculation feels imminent) is most helpful. Learn to identify the phases of ejaculation. This emission phase occurs when the semen enters the urethra and it feels as if ejaculation will occur whether stimulation continues or not. Stopping your thrusting movements will automatically reduce excitement during the preejaculatory period, thereby delaying ejaculation.

There are also pressure points on the penis just below the head on either side of the ridge (top and bottom) and at the base of the shaft next to the body (top and bottom). Applying a few seconds of continuous, firm pressure to either sets of these points can delay ejaculation if done before the point of inevitable ejaculation. Practice to see what works for you.

Being able to identify the various phases of ejaculation will improve your sense of control and confidence in your own ability to enjoy lovemaking. When you begin to feel performance anxiety or that ejaculation is imminent, try to focus on something personal about your mate. Focus on her eyes, a birthmark, the look on her face—anything but your performance. (For additional reading, see *Masters and Johnson on Sex and Human Loving*, Boston: Little, Brown and Company, 1985.)

A final note on sexuality and infertility: Therapists report that the process of rediscovering each other sexually can be a long haul for many infertile couples. They experience what happens to their sense of sexuality as a major loss. Many couples turn these feelings around after the infertility battles, but some do not. A sensitive, qualified therapist may be able to help.

AN IMPORTANT THING YOU CAN DO

Try to reintroduce yourselves to loving sensuality. Infertility can push intimacy into a secondary position in a relationship. Remember that you are friends and lovers, not just baby-makers.

#47

TAKE A VACATION FROM TRYING TO CONCEIVE

The longer you are involved with finding an infertility solution, the more changes and rough spots you are likely to encounter. Not all spouses are at the same stage at the same time. It is likely that you and your partner will be out of emotional sync as time goes on.

Infertile couples can become so focused on their separate concerns that they sometimes forget to touch base with their mates. The goal of pregnancy that they have in common is presumed by each partner to be of equal importance to the other, often to the unwitting detriment of other aspects of life. It is also possible that something is going on with your mate that you are unaware of, such as a desire to stop pursuing solutions and to look at other options.

Infertile couples often find it hard to stop pursuing solutions. They are too often pressured into "one more try" by well-meaning friends, would-be grandparents, enthusiastic doctors, new promising techniques, and each other. But there will come a time to determine when "enough is enough," and to move on to other ways to become parents or to adjust to childfree living in a positive way.

It is important to preserve the joy and intimacy in your relationship beyond the all-too-consuming quest for pregnancy. For many couples, one way to get back in touch with each other is to take a vacation from trying to conceive during some cycles. Some people combine this break with a literal vacation away from home, as well as from ovulation kits and medical practitioners. Some even use birth control methods in order to be really unplugged from pregnancy pursuits, although the hardest part of using birth control at this stage seems to be the thought that *this* would have been *the* time.

Couples report finding this vacation a real relief. It usually accomplishes one of two things. It can replenish both of you so that you have a renewed vitality with which to return to treatment, or it highlights the contrast between the burdens of treatment cycles and the ease of normal living so thoroughly that you will want to set a deadline for stopping medical solutions altogether. Either way, a vacation will help you and your mate define yourselves in relation to infertility plans.

The concepts and approaches to this phase of the infertility experience (contained in #47 through #50) were developed jointly by Merle Bombardieri, a clinical social worker and psychotherapist in Lexington, Massachusetts, and Diane Clapp, BSN, RN, a medical information counselor at the national headquarters of Resolve, Inc., who is also in private practice at Fertility Resources in Lexington, Massachusetts. Ms. Clapp is also the medical editor for Resolve's newsletter. Both have published extensively on infertility issues and are recognized authorities on the subject.

AN IMPORTANT THING YOU CAN DO

When you feel sick and tired of the whole business, take a "vacation from trying." Touch base with each other again in a way that leaves infertility out of the picture. Consider a weekend away together. Even use birth control methods for a real "time out."

#48

UNDERSTAND YOUR AMBIVALENCE

Couples can become mired in ambivalence about stopping pregnancy pursuits or continuing to endlessly try to create a child. There may always be a part of you that wants to continue, as well as a part that is fed up with the whole business. It is important to maintain an inner awareness of these opposing aspects of yourself and to attempt, at any given stage in this process, to hear which is the stronger voice.

It is also important to know that nothing is written in stone. Just because you want to put your energies into something else does not exclude trying again in the future. Even temporarily stopping doesn't mean you are a quitter, or that you weren't serious in the first place. That attitude is a way of being mean to yourself and your mate. Give yourselves credit for what you've already attempted.

One exercise to help resolve ambivalence was adapted by Merle Bombardieri from Gestalt therapy, which emphasizes resolving and integrating opposing parts of yourself. It's called "the empty chair technique," and although it may seem awkward at first, some illuminating insights often come from it. Ms. Bombardieri recommends an approach something like this:

Place two chairs opposite each other in a quiet, private room. Do not include your spouse at first. You need to hear the opposing sides of yourself in a completely free and unedited way. Designate each chair for opposite views: one for "stopping," the other for "keep on trying." Is there a part of you that feels stronger about the subject? Can you more easily imagine the dialogue from one chair than the other? If the answer is yes, then that will determine which chair to sit in first. If the answer is no, then either chair will do.

Sit in the first chair and speak for that person's viewpoint. Speak until that person is finished. Then go over to the other chair and do the same thing until that person has said everything that wants to be said. Go back and forth until you feel there is no more to say. Each side should try to convince the other. You will hear everything from demanding criticism and abuse to pleading and bargaining. That's normal. It's also normal to remain unresolved in your first several attempts.

The purpose of chair dialogues is to acquaint you with your opposing voices and to gain insight. Sometimes bargaining helps you to understand better how you feel. For instance, the "stop" voice may want "three more cycles of trying" or additional reassurance from your spouse that it's really OK to stop. But be on the lookout for the integrative voice, the one that says you do not have to produce a child to justify your existence, that you have a right to be here even if you never conceive. This compassionate voice will help you with coping and decision making, even if you decide to keep pursuing medical solutions for another year or two.

AN IMPORTANT THING YOU CAN DO

If you are bogged down with ambivalence about continuing to pursue infertility solutions, try an empty chair dialogue to help determine which is the stronger inclination in you. Understanding that ambivalence is a natural part of the process in both partners can help dissipate the paralyzing feelings that accompany ambivalence.

#49

DECIDE WHEN ENOUGH IS ENOUGH

Someday you will decide that you can no longer tolerate endless treatments and disruptions to your everyday life. You will want to put your efforts into trying something else like adoption or childfree living.

Merle Bombardieri and Diane Clapp developed a checklist to help you determine how close you are to that day. Use the list at different points in time and compare your answers with your partner's to see your attitudes as they evolve. You and your spouse should do the list separately and use different sheets of paper each time so as not to be distracted with previous answers.

Some signs that you may be ready to stop pursuing infertility solutions include:

____ Feeling "stuck" for many months; feeling that the treatment you are undergoing is futile.

____ Feeling more fed up than ever with temperature charts and urine test kits.

_____ Feeling resentful and lacking energy on the days you have doctors appointments.

_____ Realizing that you'd be disappointed if your doctor came up with a new treatment idea because you think a number of months of that treatment would just prolong your agony.

_____ Feeling that you've invested about as much time, energy, and money on infertility as you can stand; feeling that getting on with your life is more important than endlessly pursuing pregnancy.

_____ Fantasizing that your doctor or spouse suggests quitting, and you like that better than continuing to try.

_____ Beginning to fantasize, or actually talking to your doctor or spouse, about setting a deadline for stopping.

_____ Feeling that being a parent is more important at this point than how you get the baby.

_____ Feeling that you and your spouse have already mourned the loss of a biological child.

Sometimes it's difficult to tell if a stop-decision is real. People can discover areas of fear they didn't know existed. It is not unusual for people to be simultaneously afraid of parenting *and* childlessness. It's important to know that nothing is written in stone and that no one will (or should) jump out of the woodwork and accuse you of inconsistency should you decide to try a new approach after a stop-decision has been made. It's a question of what works for you, and no two couples are alike, even though many stages of infertility have common aspects.

Sometimes a new treatment or surgical method may sound promising and you might want to give it a try. You may decide that an alternative to adhering to a deadline is to live with a time frame instead. A time frame does not state how many cycles you will attempt to endure multiple procedures. A time frame puts brackets around a period of time beyond which you will go back to your stop-decision. For example, you may decide to try a specific approach for one year and no longer; or it can be an age-related time frame beyond which you will not go. That's a way of honoring the very real stop-decision that you've made, while keeping the door cracked on something new. Sometimes a stop-decision actually turns out to be just a vacation from trying, and you may discover renewed determination to continue. But often a stop-decision is just that and you know it in your heart. Even *then* you may be tempted into something new, and it's important to allow yourselves the option to try.

Many couples who adopt children actually incorporate various approaches for subsequent biological children. Sometimes couples with male infertility (like low sperm counts) decide to try artificial donor insemination for a first child and to explore other methods using the husband's sperm later on.

Some couples feel that biological children are the only avenue they care to pursue, while others feel that parenting itself is their main goal. There are a number of approaches and options. The trick is to discover what is best for you both.

There are crucial stages that must receive personal attention, otherwise ambivalence and sometimes unprocessed rage can be carried over into new decisions. For instance a man who hasn't adequately dealt with the fact that he will not be a biological father may unconsciously resent children conceived through donor sperm and subtly withdraw from the family. Women who haven't dealt with the issue of not being able to bear a child may subtly resent adopted children.

It is tough to avoid feeling any of these emotions because they are not inappropriate for the circumstances. But it is important not to let them fester and undermine your happiness in covert ways. A good infertility therapist will help you continue to grow through the stages that inevitably occur with infertility.

Many couples choose to remain childfree. After giving conception their best shot, many people feel battle-weary and sometimes report feeling a loss of innocence. But these feelings fade as couples renew, rekindle, and rediscover the time when they were happy together—before they were even aware of their infertility. They turn their attention back to the things that engaged them before, or develop new interests based on what they have come to learn about themselves. It is not easy to relinquish a dream held in common, but it can be done.

AN IMPORTANT THING YOU CAN DO

Give yourselves credit for the incredible effort you've made. Begin to turn your attention to the future.

#50

PAY GENTLE ATTENTION TO GRIEF AND MOURNING

In the infertile world, effort does not guarantee success. Before moving on, you have to grieve what didn't happen *as a couple*. Depending on the cause of the infertility, this process will be different for each partner and can have several components, such as mourning the loss of genetic continuity or the loss of the pregnancy process itself. In fact, moving on to another alternative too quickly may be an avoidance of essential grief work.

It's common for infertile couples to process about 70 percent of their grief and to keep about 30 percent locked into the continuing hope for pregnancy. Couples who have done a significant amount of grieving may be surprised by the intense anger, regret, and sadness that well up when they decide to stop trying. For those who have done little or no grieving, the reaction to ceasing their efforts may be even more extreme.

There are two kinds of "knowing" that pregnancy will not occur. There is the intellectual knowing, and allowing yourselves some feelings about it. And then there's knowing it in your heart of hearts. Many people don't fully grasp this loss until they make an absolute decision to stop trying. Many people attempt to avoid grief by grasping at straws, searching for new doctors and different medical treatments. A sudden desperate attempt at pregnancy after a decision to stop trying may be a refusal to grieve.

It's not unusual for these feelings to well up within the first few weeks of a stop-decision. Try not to judge yourselves too harshly. Reassure yourselves that if the decision truly turns out to be not what you want, you can always go back to trying.

Chances are, however, that after some more time to mourn and to get used to the idea of the stop-decision, you won't want to start up again. Within a short time you will be enjoying the relief of no longer having to strive so hard, as well as enjoying the added time, energy, and attention you have for other things, including exploring alternative routes, such as adoption, if you so choose, or childfree living, with all its accompanying possibilities.

AN IMPORTANT THING YOU CAN DO

Allow as much time as you need to grieve and mourn what has not happened. Be gentle and loving with yourself and with your partner. Begin gradually to inform family members and friends. Many couples come to understand, after a period of rage and mourning, that infertility is not the end of the world but rather the presentation of different opportunities and completely new beginnings.

INDEX